Essential Clinical Social Work Series

Series Editor

Carol Tosone, School of Social Work, New York University, New York, NY, USA

More information about this series at http://www.springer.com/series/8115

Gillian O'Shea Brown

Healing Complex Posttraumatic Stress Disorder

A Clinician's Guide

Springer

Gillian O'Shea Brown
New York University
New York, NY, USA

ISSN 2520-162X ISSN 2520-1611 (electronic)
Essential Clinical Social Work Series
ISBN 978-3-030-61415-7 ISBN 978-3-030-61416-4 (eBook)
https://doi.org/10.1007/978-3-030-61416-4

This Springer imprint is published by the registered company Springer Nature Switzerland AG
The registered company address is: Gewerbestrasse 11, 6330 Cham, Switzerland

To my husband, Grant Elgin Brown,
I am a firm believer that if just one person believes in you with the conviction that you can triumph – all things are possible. You have always given me the wings to fly and a safe space to land. Thank you for championing me and never questioning my relentless dreaming, no matter how bizarre. I dedicate this book to you.

Acknowledgments

There are so many people to whom I owe a debt of gratitude for their assistance and support as I worked on this book. However, firstly, I must thank my clients both past and present. Bearing witness to their stories and lived experiences has been by far my greatest honor and learning experience. Moments of awe, resonance, and compassion have motivated me to continue to train, seek new knowledge, and grow professionally, so that I could serve in a way that feels meaningful and impactful. I did not set out to become a trauma therapist; however, those who presented themselves to me had all walked on the pathway of trauma. It became apparent to me early in my career that to serve as a healer of trauma, I would need to expand my toolbox and my knowledge base. It has been my honor to witness so many people's healing journeys. I write this book in the hope that I can share what I have learnt so far. However, I know that I will continue to dedicate my life to deepening my knowledge in this area and sharing it with all of those whose lives have been touched by trauma.

I would like to thank Carol Tosone, PhD, the editor of the *Essential Clinical Social Work* Series. She has served as a professional mentor and friend to me over the past few years, as well as serving as chair of my doctoral committee. There are certain people that cross your path in life, and through their relentless persistence, they forge change and growth – whether you're ready for it or not. Jung says there are no mistakes, only synchronicities – I am deeply grateful for this serendipitous union for many reasons. I first spoke with Dr. Tosone in 2016 when I applied for a doctoral program at New York University. I deferred my acceptance as I weighed the pros and cons to such a life commitment. However, her conviction in me and gentle guidance spurred me on, to accept and proceed. Later she convinced me to write this book. She is the kind of person that can direct you with such persuasion that you forget all of the excuses that held you back before the conversation. I have yet to find the terminology to explain this particular skill set – but it exists within her. She is truly the trauma queen.

I would also like to extend my sincere gratitude to Ayan Mukherjee for his generous contribution to this book. Ayan kindly permitted to have his illustrations included in this book. Ayan is a psychotherapist who creates mental health art for psychoeducational purposes. To learn more please visit his website: www.therapyillustrated.com. I would like to thank Janet Kim, MPH, of Springer for her unceasing support throughout the process. The extent of her diligence and patience are rare professional attributes, and I am grateful that I have benefited from her time and effort. I have been fortunate enough to have many wonderful professional mentors over the course of my career, including Eileen Hogan, PhD; Kenneth Burns, PhD; Brid Kiely, MSW; Lavina Temple, BSW; Beverli Mormile, PsyD; Sarah St. Onge, PhD; Lydia Denton, LCSW; Elizabeth Janssen, NP; Greg Carson, LCSW and Deany Laliotis, LICSW. Their insights, knowledge, and compassionate lens in the field of trauma have expanded my clinical understanding greatly. I would like to thank Elizabeth Janssen, NP, for her rich contribution to Chapter 9 of this book, which details ego states and inner child work. Through her background in psychoanalytic theory, eye movement desensitization and reprocessing (EMDR), and internal family systems (IFS), she has an intimate knowledge of the anatomy of trauma. Elizabeth served as my clinical supervisor at Integrative Trauma Program at the National Institute for the Psychotherapies; her passion and wide repertoire of clinical knowledge always kept me intrigued and stimulated during our time together. I would like to dedicate Chapter 7, which focuses on beliefs, to Lydia Denton, LCSW, another past clinical supervisor. She educated me on the power of belief and introduced me to the works of Bruce Lipton and Michael A. Singer. She sparks playfulness, joy, and inspiration into every room she graces with her worldly presence.

I would like to thank my colleagues and peers who graciously offered to proofread chapters: Aviva Glass, PhD; Elizabeth Janssen, NP; and Rachelle Kammer, PhD. I would like to thank Tyler Hancock for his vision, patience and keen eye for detail. I would like to thank my doctoral cohort at New York University for their peer support, encouragement, and humor. Listed alphabetically: Terry Audate, Marina Angela Badillo, Constance Catrone, Jessica Chock Goldman, Jasmine Collazo, Angelique Cortez, Anne Dempsey, Maddy Ellberger, Max Kusovitsky, Stacey Gordan, Nick Santo, and Dayna Sedillo-Hamann. It has been an honor to share time and conversation with such brilliant minds and dedicated hearts. I would also like to thank my wonderful friends for their patience, understanding, and continuous support. Last but not least, I would like to thank my patient and supportive husband, family, and magnificent in-laws. I feel such gratitude to have so much love and support in my life. Creativity and playfulness can only occur when you feel safe; all of the above have given me the opportunity to feel held and supported in the world and for that I am eternally grateful.

Contents

About the Author

Gillian O'Shea Brown LCSW, DSW, is an Irish born psychotherapist and EMDRIA-certified therapist. Dr. O'Shea Brown has trained at University College Cork, New York University and the National Institute for the Psychotherapies. She currently serves as adjunct faculty at NYU and maintains a private practice in Manhattan, New York. She can be contacted by email: gillosheabrownlcsw@gmail.com.

List of Abbreviations

AAI	Adult Attachment Interview
AAS	Adult Attachment Scale
ACE	Adverse Childhood Experiences
ACES	Adverse Childhood Experiences Study
ACE-Q	Adverse Childhood Experiences Questionnaire
AIP	Adaptive Information Processing
APA	American Psychiatric Association
ASD	Acute Stress Disorder
BAA	Business Associate Agreement
BPD	Borderline Personality Disorder
CC	Corpus Callosum
CDC	The Centers for Disease Control and Prevention
COVID	"CO" stands for "corona," "VI" for "virus," and "D" for "disease"
C-PTSD	Complex Posttraumatic Stress Disorder
DSM	The Diagnostic and Statistical Manual of Mental Disorders
EMDR	Eye Movement Desensitization and Reprocessing
EMDRIA	Eye Movement Desensitization and Reprocessing International Association
FCC	Federal Communications Commission
FDA	Food and Drug Administration
DES-II	Scale of Dissociative Experiences II
DID	Dissociative Identity Disorder
EBP	Evidence-Based Practice
HIPAA	Health Insurance Portability and Accountability Act
ICD	11 International Classifications of Diseases, 11th Revision
IFS	Internal Family Systems
IPV	Intimate Partner Violence
ITQ	International Trauma Questionnaire
PG	Posttraumatic Growth
SRT	Shame Resilience Theory

PTSD	Posttraumatic Stress Disorder
SE	Somatic Experiencing
SP	Sensorimotor Psychotherapy
TF-CBT	Trauma Focused Cognitive Behavioral Therapy
WHO	World Health Organization
PCL-5	The PTSD Checklist for DSM-5
RDI	Resource Development and Installation
REM	Rapid Eye Movement
mHealth Apps	Mobile Health Applications
VEMDR	Virtual Eye Movement Desensitization and Reprocessing

Chapter 1
Introduction

The word trauma is derived from the Greek word "wound," which can refer to wounds of either a physical or psychological nature. The term "complex trauma" is used to describe chronic traumatization, for instance, the experience of multiple and/or prolonged developmentally adverse traumatic events, most often of an interpersonal nature. Complex trauma is the result of chronic, prolonged, and repeated trauma arising from childhood abuse, neglect, and/or exposure to domestic violence. Survivors of complex relational trauma often present as consumed with shame, distrustful, and actively wounded, years or even decades after their so-called escape to freedom. Judith Herman, MD, was one of the first to differentiate the unique experience of complex trauma from single incident trauma:

> *Many abused children cling to the hope that growing up will bring escape and freedom... But the personality formed in the environment of coercive control is not well adapted to adult life. The survivor is left with fundamental problems in basic trust, autonomy, and initiative... [As an adult, the survivor is] burdened by major impairments in self-care, in cognition and in memory, in identity, and in the capacity to form stable relationships. [Survivors remain] prisoners of childhood, attempting to create a new life, [but still] reencountering the trauma.* (Herman, 1992a, p.80)

Herman (1992a) researched the residual impacts of complex trauma on vulnerability, identity, and experiences within relationships.

Complex trauma is insidious and pervasive in our society; it changes the way an individual perceives themselves and others, in addition to adversely impacting how safe and secure one feels in navigating the world around them. After decades of diligent effort from Herman (1992b), van der Kolk, McFarlane, and Weisaeth (1996), and others, complex trauma is just now coming to prominence. Complex posttraumatic stress disorder (C-PTSD) is a diagnostic entity included in the *International Classification of Diseases, 11th revision* (*ICD-11*). Endorsement of the *ICD-11* definition of C-PTSD will come into effect on January 1, 2022. C-PTSD denotes a severe form of PTSD that is the result of prolonged and repeated trauma. Therefore, healing complex trauma can prove to be a challenging and complicated process.

G. O'Shea Brown, *Healing Complex Posttraumatic Stress Disorder*, Essential Clinical Social Work Series, https://doi.org/10.1007/978-3-030-61416-4_1

People are often less willing to talk about problems that they believe others do not have, which contributes to a particular veil of shame and secrecy that surrounds complex trauma. After many years of walking on eggshells, the silence and secrecy can grow familiar, like an old friend. Survivors may surmise that others will not understand or may unfairly pass judgment or blame regarding their trauma history. In our profession, we are deeply privileged to witness so many people's healing journeys. This book is a clinician's guide to understanding, diagnosing, treating, and healing C-PTSD. It provides guidance on healing complex trauma through phase-oriented, multimodal, and skill-focused treatment approaches, with a core emphasis on symptom relief and functional improvement.

By reading this book, you will become more familiar with the integrative healing techniques and modalities that are currently being utilized as evidence-based treatments. In addition, you will develop a language for, understanding of, and deeper compassion toward the pain you are witnessing. This book provides a fresh theoretical perspective regarding diathetic factors in the development of C-PTSD, in addition to interweaving psychoanalytic theory, neuroscience, and contemporary integrative techniques into clinical practice. The clinical guidance shared in this book can be applied in a full range of clinical practice settings, with adults and families in both private practice and diverse agency settings.

To understand the imprint of complex trauma, the foundational step is to earn the trust of the survivor. From there we can begin to provide them with the knowledge, psychoeducation, and terminology to understand what they have survived, and in doing so, we strive to create for them a place of safety, something they may never have experienced in those painful formative years. This book also explores a broad range of evidence-based treatments through literature review and clinical vignettes. Posttraumatic growth and resilience shall also be critically reviewed from a theoretical and clinical lens.

As part of the introduction to this book, I would like to address the title. It is my intention that the word "healing" will instill a sense of optimism and hope to those who recognize the impacts of deep relational trauma wounds. When a client privileges you by expressing their pain, this is a sign of healing. When a client shows up each week, courageous, open, and willing, this is a sign of healing. When a client advocates for themselves by saying that they are feeling unsafe or untrusting of the process, this, too, is a sign of healing. Healing is an ever-unfolding process of evolution, vulnerability, and self-compassion. Healing is a continuous process of learning to choose: choosing yourself, choosing a better life, and, most importantly, choosing self-care over self-destruction. Healing is a process of unburdening, becoming more yourself, and becoming more than you could have ever hoped for in your darkest and most ominous moments. Healing allows a client to operate out of deep self-awareness rather than classic conditioning. Freud said we repeat rather than remember. At times, we witness our clients relive, re-experience, or even reenact their pain many times over. In the words of Herman (1992a), "the resolution of the trauma is never final; recovery is never complete" (p.152). The impact of past traumatic events may be awakened at particular points, despite being sufficiently resolved at one stage of recovery in the life cycle. Though we as clinicians cannot always take the pain away, we can take that walk with them, serving as their empathic witness and guide as they work to overcome these milestones in the healing journey.

I suggest reading each chapter in order, as the knowledge you gain in each chapter serves as a foundation for the next. Following each chapter, there will be brief study questions and class exercises for professors and students using this book as a textbook in their graduate school classes. In service of brevity, this book provides a broad base of foundational knowledge; however, this book does not serve as a substitute for trauma-informed clinical training and certification. Reviewing the Appendix will provide guidance on deepening your clinical knowledge and practice as part of continuous professional development.

Chapter 2 provides an exploration of attachment theory with a description of each of the adult attachment categories, in addition to outlining the role of attunement and mirroring. This chapter will review current research on the implications of insecure attachment for adult relationships and social functioning. Following this overview, a critique of attachment theory shall be considered. Subsequently, an exploration of how COVID-19 has exacerbated the impact of developmental trauma shall be critically reviewed. Finally, the chapter will briefly introduce interventions utilized to measure adult attachment status in a clinical setting. This is intended to familiarize you with the measurement of attachment, and it is not a replacement for the clinical training to administer such measurements.

Chapter 3 provides an overview of the emergence of complex posttraumatic stress disorder (C-PTSD), including an overview of symptoms and an explanation of how C-PTSD is unique from other diagnoses. The chapter examines insecure attachment and relational trauma as diathetic factors in the development of C-PTSD. Following this overview, the neuroscience of complex trauma, with specific attention to the mind-body connection, will be critically explored. Subsequently, this chapter will present a measurement tool utilized to assess the impact of trauma in a clinical setting. Once again, you will be provided with foundational knowledge and guidance on how to measure trauma symptoms; however, trauma-focused training and certification is strongly advised.

Chapter 4 will provide a description of what constitutes a dysfunctional family system before exploring how dysfunction can lead to pathological accommodation. The role of communication deviance and behavioral abnormalities within the family system shall be reviewed, and this chapter will evaluate current research exploring the impact that adverse childhood experiences (ACEs) have on identity, adult relationships, and social functioning. Finally, the chapter will explore how dysfunction within a family system can be measured using the ACE Questionnaire as a clinical tool.

Chapter 5 will provide a description of the role, purpose, and function of dissociation from a trauma-informed perspective. The chapter will explore how dissociative experiencing can be measured within a clinical setting, utilizing the Scale of Dissociative Experiences II. Following this review of the clinical tool, this chapter explores the signs and symptoms of dissociation before considering the practice implications of working with dissociative clients. Finally, strategies to orient a client to the present moment shall be illustrated via clinical vignette.

The foundation of trauma healing begins with locating a sense of safety in the body, in addition to enhancing the survivor's awareness and knowledge about the body's responses to trauma. This allows a client to operate out of deep self-awareness rather than classic conditioning. Chapter 6 begins by providing an overview of the how trauma impacts the mind and body. Second, the significance of affective states will be reviewed through the lens of the Modulation Model and Polyvagal Theory. This chapter will explore the concepts of implicit memory and somatization in the context of complex trauma treatment. Finally, this chapter will review the existing relevant literature exploring the relationship between chronic stress and immune system impairment.

Experiences create thoughts, which become metabolized into memory, perception, and identity. Beliefs become stronger and even more deeply rooted when they are repeatedly affirmed by our environment. Chapter 7 will begin by reviewing how core negative beliefs form in the unconscious mind before reviewing the role that bias plays in shaping an individual's perceptions of reality. Subsequently this chapter will explore how beliefs contribute to the psychological phenomenon in which individuals may have an inclination to reenact traumatic or painful events; how beliefs impact experiences in close relationships will also be considered. Finally, this chapter will review how blocking beliefs can be linked to memories from which they are formed, in addition to exploring how self-determination impacts the clinical process.

The field of psychotherapy has increasingly become influenced by evidence-based practice (EBP), which is centered on the ethos of research-informed practice and practice-informed research. Consequently, treatment planning and the clinical decision-making process are informed by best practice guidelines developed from research findings. Complex trauma treatment has evolved into a more integrative, body-oriented approach. Chapter 8 will first provide an overview of Trauma-Focused Cognitive Behavioral Therapy as a psychotherapy modality for treating complex trauma. Second, an outline of the process of Eye Movement Desensitization and Reprocessing therapy will be offered. Subsequently, a review of the benefits of body-based therapies such as Sensorimotor Psychotherapy and Somatic Experiencing in treating complex trauma shall be discussed. Finally, this chapter shall discuss the implications for psychotherapy arising from COVID-19—more specifically, the fact that virtual therapy has gone from being an emerging trend in clinical practice to a necessary adaptation during COVID-19 (O'Shea Brown, 2021).

A multi-consciousness approach to clinical treatment enables the trauma survivor to hear from the various parts of the consciousness through a compassionate lens which can ultimately pave the way for negotiation, clarity, and inner harmony. Thoughtful application of ego-state-informed language can facilitate compassionate nonjudgmental witnessing of the parts that are coming to voice so that they can be heard and even unburdened of their fears. Chapter 9 will begin by exploring the relationship between trauma and the multiplicity of the mind, illustrated through clinical vignette. An overview of the theoretical underpinning and application of the Internal Family Systems Model will be provided.

Through my observations of my clients, I have witnessed the undeniable power of resilience, that is, the ability that humans have to adapt to, navigate, and even grow from life's most painful events. Resilience has been described as the capacity to adapt successfully to disturbances that threaten functioning, sustainability, and future development. Therefore, resilience is not the absence of suffering but the capacity to adapt to survive in painful or unpredictable circumstances. Researchers have even argued that survival through hardship and triumph over adversity can make a survivor more focused and more feeling and, in turn, expand one's capacity for compassion, spirituality, and creativity (Brown, 2006; Garmezy, 1993; Garmezy & Masten, 1986; Miller, 1997; Sapienza & Masten, 2011; Scheff, 2003). Chapter 10 begins with an exploration of vulnerability and shame through the lens of Shame Resilience Theory (Brown, 2006). Subsequently, the anatomy of resilience will be explored through a theoretical and clinical lens. Finally, this chapter will explore the emergence and impact of the Posttraumatic Growth Model and the impact this has on an individual's intuition, internal guidance, and power.

Shared trauma in the wake of a global pandemic has created a unique bond between the clinician and the client. While navigating one's own fears, anxieties, and losses, the clinician must also serve as an anchor to the client in an unsteady and unpredictable world. The profound impact of collective catastrophic events can create immense hardship for clinicians living and working in traumatogenic environments. Even outside of the pandemic, clinicians who specialize in the treatment of trauma and complex trauma have a distinct susceptibility to vicarious trauma (VT) due to the repeated exposure to the harrowing details of their clients' traumatic experiences. VT refers to the experience of indirect trauma such as the clinicians' continuous emotional engagement with a clients' traumatic material. This can create cognitive distortions and changes in the core belief system of the clinician, which, in turn, can adversely impact overall functioning and emotional well-being. Many clinicians enter into the profession to compassionately witness, heal, and affirm their clients due to their own lived experiences of trauma. Without adequate use of clinical supervision, professional boundaries, and self-care, repeated exposure to trauma can be precarious to the clinician's well-being, causing retraumatization or compassion fatigue. Chapter 11 will provide a conceptualization of VT, before exploring how this may impact upon the clinician and the therapeutic alliance. Secondly, this chapter will review the impact of countertransference before proposing strategies to effectively manage its adverse effects. Finally, this chapter will explore the role of professional supervision and the importance of self-care for the trauma clinician. To conclude, in Chapter 12, this book will reflect on the topics explored in addition to discussing visions for the future of practice in terms of treating, healing, and preventing complex trauma.

References

Brown, B. (2006). Shame resilience theory: A grounded theory of women and shame. *Families in Society, 87*(01).

Garmezy, N. (1993). Vulnerability and resilience. In D. C. Funder, R. D. Parke, et al. (Eds.), *Studying lives through time: Personality and development* (pp. 377–398). Washington, DC: American Psychological Association.

Garmezy, N., & Masten, A. S. (1986). Stress, competence, and resilience: Common frontiers for therapist and psychopathologist. *Behavior Therapy, 17*(5), 500.

Herman, J. L. (1992a). *Trauma and recovery: The aftermath of violence*. New York, NY: Basic Books.

Herman, J. L. (1992b). Complex PTSD: A syndrome in survivors of prolonged and repeated trauma. *Journal of Traumatic Stress, 5*(3), 377–391. https://doi.org/10.1002/jts.2490050305

Miller, A. (1997). *Drama of the gifted child: The search for the true self.* New York, NY: Basic Books.

O'Shea Brown, G. (2021). Reflections on providing virtual eye movement desensitization and reprocessing therapy in the wake of COVID-19: Survival through adaptation. In C. Tosone (Ed.), *Shared trauma, shared resilience during a pandemic: Social work in the time of COVID-19*. Cham, Switzerland: Springer.

Sapienza, J. K., & Masten, A. S. (2011). Understanding and promoting resilience in children and youth. *Current Opinion in Psychiatry, 24*(4), 267–273. https://doi.org/10.1097/YCO.0b013e32834776a8

Scheff, T. (2003). Shame in self and society. *Symbolic Interaction, 26*, 239–262.

van der Kolk, B. A., McFarlane, A., & Weisaeth, L. (1996). *Traumatic stress*. New York, NY: Guilford Press.

Chapter 2
Understanding Your Emotional Map

Our early experiences with attachment figures set a precedent not just for the development of a sense of self but also for the development of healthy relationships later in life. A secure attachment is formed when caregivers are stable, reliable, and trustworthy in their behaviors and responsivity (Bowlby, 1973). Bowlby (1989) hypothesized that a child's earliest experiences with their parents lead to the development of beliefs regarding self-worth, safety, and security and the trustworthiness of others, which he termed the *internal working model.* Children make sense of the world by creating emotional maps to assist them in discerning who they should trust and how they will survive. When children's needs are adequately met, they can begin to develop trust that the world is an intrinsically benevolent place. However, in the event of pervasive relational trauma in childhood, such as persistent patterns of rejection, humiliation, or neglect, children can develop an insecure or disorganized attachment with a caregiver. The insecure attachment can negatively affect their ability to establish a sense of safety and maintain healthy relationships, which interferes with their future capacity to parent effectively or trust relationally (Lee & Hankin, 2009; Main & Hesse, 1990; van IJzendoorn, 1995). Furthermore, an insecure attachment pattern may serve as a vulnerability factor for adversity in adulthood (Bowlby, 1973).

This chapter will first provide an exploration of attachment theory, including a description of each of the adult attachment categories, in addition to outlining the role of attunement and mirroring in building attachment. It will then review current research on the implications of insecure attachment for adult relationships and social functioning. Following this overview, a critique of attachment theory shall be considered. Subsequently, an exploration of how COVID-19 has exacerbated the impact of developmental trauma shall be offered. Finally, the chapter will briefly introduce interventions utilized to measure adult attachment patterns in a clinical setting.

G. O'Shea Brown, *Healing Complex Posttraumatic Stress Disorder*, Essential Clinical Social Work Series, https://doi.org/10.1007/978-3-030-61416-4_2

Attachment, Attunement, and Mirroring: An Overview

Bowlby first sought to understand a child's connection to their preferred object or caregiver, as an attachment figure. The attachment figure serves a dual purpose: providing a secure base from which a child can explore and serving as a source of comfort when needed (Bowlby, 1973). An optimal attachment figure is characterized as stable, responsive, and trustworthy, thereby forming a secure attachment pattern (Bowlby, 1980). Conversely, when attachment figures are unstable, unpredictable, or untrustworthy, this results in the development of an insecure attachment pattern (Bowlby, 1973). Ainsworth first introduced the Strange Situation paradigm as an empirical measure to assess mother-infant attachment status between 18-month-old infants and their mothers as a means to observe and assess the parent-infant attachment pattern.

The Strange Situation assessment is comprised of the child's brief separation from their primary caregiver and subsequent reunion (see Table 2.1). Importantly, reflecting the culture of the period, this study only represented mothers as primary caregivers. This assessment procedure simulated the naturalistic stress experienced by infants following the disappearance of their primary caregiver, under the assumption that the caregiver will return again to resume care (Ainsworth & Bell, 1970). Ainsworth identified three main attachment patterns on the basis of the infants' behaviors following the separation and reunion procedure: secure, anxious-avoidant, and anxious-ambivalent. Later Ainsworth expanded the categories to include disorganized (unclassifiable) as proposed by Main and Solomon (1990). An infant's responses to separation and reunification provide insight into the quality of their attachment with their caregiver and reveal developmental changes in the infant's coping strategies and self-regulation. In the Strange Situation, the securely attached infants became emotionally distressed following the parent's departure and appeared

Table 2.1 Attachment patterns and the respective behaviors associated with each during the "Strange Situation experiment"

Attachment pattern	Exploration/ orientation toward parent	Behavior when parents exit the room	Stranger anxiety	Behavior in response to reunion	Parent's behavior
Secure	Explores unfamiliar room with an orientation toward parent	Some discomfort	Comfortable with stranger when parent is present	Greeted parent positively	Sensitive, supportive, and attuned
Anxious-ambivalent (Insecure)	No orientation to parent when exploring the room	Unconcerned about parent's absence	Comfortable with stranger	Uninterested	Misattunement, rejection (ignoring infant)
Anxious-avoidant (Insecure)	Unconcerned about exploring the room	Intense distress	Uncomfortable with stranger	Rejected parent	Inconsistent

to be emotionally comforted upon reunification (Ainsworth, 1967). Infants with a secure attachment explored the environment with an orientation toward the parent. When the parent exited the room, the securely attached infant expressed some discomfort. Infants with an anxious-avoidant attachment did not explore the environment, regardless of who was present, and avoided or ignored the parent upon their return. These anxious-avoidant infants did not outwardly exhibit distress when the parent left or when the parent returned; instead they internalized and masked their true emotion. Anxious-ambivalent infants did not demonstrate outward distress at separation. Upon reunification with the parent, anxious-ambivalent infants presented as clingy but simultaneously resistant to comfort from the parent (Ainsworth & Bell, 1970). Infants in this category demonstrated signs of resentment in response to the absence and helpless passivity.

The final category of insecure attachment pattern, which was later added to Ainsworth's classification system, is disorganized attachment. Disorganized attachment is applied to infant attachment patterns as described by Main and Solomon, which were deemed unclassifiable with respect to Ainsworth's classification system (1986). Disorganized attachment patterns are characterized by a lack of coordinated behaviors in line with other attachment patterns; the infant with a disorganized attachment pattern will display signs of disorientation, confusion, or fear of the parent (George & Solomon, 2011; Main & Solomon, 1986). Disorganized infant attachment patterns are most common in those who have endured neglect/child abuse, and this category accounts for approximately 15% of cases in normative samples (Lyons-Ruth & Jacobvitz, 2008). Main and Hesse (1990) assert the hypothesis that if the parent arouses the infant's fear, this will place the infant in an unresolvable paradox regarding whether to approach the parent for comfort. The disorganized attachment behaviors of infants are gradually replaced by controlling strategies referred to as controlling-punitive and controlling-caregiving. The controlling subgroups superficially present as more organized; controlling behavior usually takes the form of a punitive or caregiving with respect to the parent (Main & Cassidy, 1988; Solomon, George, & De Jong, 1995). Controlling-punitive behavior is characterized by the child's attempts to maintain the parent's attention and engagement through hostile, coercive, or more subtle recruitment behaviors. Controlling-caregiving behavior is characterized by the child's attempts to maintain the parent's attention and involvement by entertaining, organizing, and/or directing the parent, as seen in the "parentified child." Both disorganized attachment strategies in infancy and controlling attachment strategies in the preschool years are associated with aggression and psychopathology (Carlson, 1998). Furthermore, disorganized attachment in infancy is predictive of higher levels of dissociative symptoms and overall psychopathology in late adolescence. The term disorganized attachment pattern is generally only utilized to refer to infants, and the terms disoriented and dysregulated are applied to describe children, adolescents, and adults in this category (George & Solomon, 2011).

A secure attachment is formed when the caregiver demonstrates sensitivity to the child's emerging intentionality through mentalizing, that is, the caregiver's ability to understand the child's inner emerging subjectivity (Fonagy, Gergely, & Target,

2007). This requires the parent to demonstrate attunement and mirroring. Relational attunement refers to the degree to which interactive partners (in this case, a parent and infant) are "in sync" and engaged in goal-directed cooperation (Bowlby, 1969/1982). Mirroring refers to an interpersonal phenomenon in which the attachment figure adjusts the timing and content of their behavioral movements such that they mirror the child's behavioral and emotional cues. This behavior fosters empathy and builds rapport (Ainsworth, 1982; Chartrand & Bargh, 1999). In 1975, Edward Tronick PhD and colleagues first presented the "Still Face Experiment," which was conducted by placing an infant face to face with their mother and directing the mother to remain non-responsive and expressionless, following 3 minutes of free interaction (Tronick, Als, Adamson, Wise, & Brazelton, 1978). After repeated attempts to engage their mother, the infant typically orients their face and body away from the mother with a withdrawn, hopeless facial expression (Tronick & Gold, 2020).

Unfortunately, this "still face" response elicited from an infant can inadvertently be replicated in the client-clinician dyad when the clinician does not mirror a client's emotional reactivity and vulnerability. This may happen in the context of misattunement or simply during telepsychotherapy impacted by poor Internet connectivity. (The timing and attunement of the therapeutic process can be adversely impacted by poor Internet connectivity and audio dysfunction. The practice implications of telepsychotherapy in the wake of COVID-19 will be discussed further in Chap. 8.) Regardless, the "still face" causes undue stress and potentially interferes with the trust-building needed to access vulnerability. Conversely, mirroring is used as a technique to attune to the client's needs through reflective listening and empathic understanding of the client's physical and emotional cues. Secure attachment experiences in both parenting and psychotherapy require mentalizing and in turn lead to the formation of epistemic trust (i.e., the individual's willingness to experience the environment and consider new information as trustworthy) (Corriveau et al., 2009). These behaviors promote the intergenerational passage of healthy relationships.

Implications of an Insecure Attachment Pattern

A past study examining the transmission of adult attachment status from one generation to another estimated that there is 70% correspondence between the mother's attachment status and the attachment status of their child (De Wolff & van IJzendoorn, 1997; Grossmann, Fremmer-Bombik, Rudolph, & Grossmann, 1988). This research hypothesized that parents with a secure attachment status are most sensitively attuned and likely to mirror their children's behavioral and emotional cues, leading to a higher likelihood of a secure attachment in their offspring. Conversely this research hypothesized that parents with an anxious-avoidant pattern, as opposed to those with a secure attachment, would more likely avoid closeness and intense emotions. Consequently, a strong expression of need from their offspring may lead to parental withdrawal (van IJzendoorn, 1992). If seeking attention leads to rejection from the non-responsive parent, the child will likely develop an avoidant attachment, inhibiting the desire to seek comfort in order to maintain physical proximity (Grossmann et al., 1988). Insecure attachment can be seen as an injury rather than a disorder, since during this pivotal time it allows the child to adapt to ensure survival in an unpredictable and/or adversarial environment.

Past work has also demonstrated that parents with an anxious-ambivalent attachment pattern become easily overwhelmed by their children's behavior (Grossman et al., 1988). Consequently, these parents demonstrated inconsistency in their ability to attune to and respond sensitively to their children's cues. The children of such attachment figures are inclined to develop an anxious-ambivalent attachment pattern, exhibiting demanding, angry behaviors as an adaptive method of attention seeking in an environment where subtlety is often overlooked (van IJzendoorn, 1995). Parents with a disorganized attachment pattern, referred to as dysregulated, are most likely to have children with disorganized attachment (Grossmann et al., 1988; van IJzendoorn, 1992). Main and Hesse (1990) postulated that parents with a dysregulated attachment status exhibit specific frightening behaviors which activates a startle response in their children. Often these parents behave this way due to their own unresolved childhood experiences, such as emotional dysregulation and psychological reactivity, which can be triggered by their children's cues. Maltreatment by parents is a direct precursor to disorganized attachment in children, with the majority of maltreated children demonstrating a disorganized attachment status (Granqvist et al., 2017).

Survivors of attachment trauma often adopt maladaptive behaviors and personality traits, in addition to developing an insecure attachment patterns (Bowlby, 1989; American Psychological Association, 2013). Furthermore, attachment disorganization in childhood is connected with problems related to dissociation and other types of pathology in adolescence and adulthood (Ainsworth, 1982). Secure attachments serve as a protective factor against toxic levels of stress and serve a critical role in the organization of the neurophysiological substrates responsible for self-regulation (Ainsworth, Blehar, Waters, & Wall, 1978; Bowlby, 1980; Hertsgaard, Gunnar, Erickson, & Nachmias, 1995; Shore, 2003). The experience of trauma in the formative years and/or maltreatment by attachment figures creates a vulnerability to severe emotional dysregulation along with intense feelings of despair, anxiety, shame, and mistrust of others later on in life (Wesselmann, 2013; Wesselmann et al., 2012). Furthermore, insecurely attached individuals' difficulty establishing affect regulation has been linked to impaired capacity to delay gratification throughout life.

The Stanford Marshmallow Experiment was a series of studies conducted to measure a child's ability to delay gratification in the 1960s–1970s. Children were placed in a room by themselves and given one edible treat with the instructions that if they could wait 15 min, they would receive a total of two edible treats. Mischel et al. (2011) found that in a sample of over 600 children, with an age range from 3 years and 6 months to 5 years and 8 months (the median age was 4 years and 6 months), approximately one third practiced delayed gratification long enough to obtain both treats. Mischel discovered through longitudinal studies that the insecurely attached infant participants of the Strange Situation were far less likely to practice delayed gratification when participating in the Marshmallow Test a few years later when compared to their securely attached peers (Mischel, 2014). The infants who were unable to activate effective coping strategies during the Strange Situation were also unable to practice delayed gratification in the Marshmallow Test. Poignantly, the longitudinal research demonstrated that the children who had not yet mastered delayed gratification in the Marshmallow Test exhibited higher levels of impulsivity and poorer emotional regulation later on. This led to higher instances of academic underachievement, poverty, poor health, and substance misuse and a higher likelihood of marriage ending in divorce (Mischel, 2014; Mischel et al., 2011; NICHD, 1998).

Insecure Attachment and Romantic Relationships

Previous literature has shown that anxious-avoidant romantic partners are characterized by fear of intimacy and anxious-ambivalent romantic partners are preoccupied with the longing for reciprocation and union (Hazan & Shaver, 1987). Compared with their securely attached peers, both insecurely attached groups self-reported higher instances of negative experiences, instability, and dissatisfaction in the context of their relationships. Collins and Read (1990) also demonstrated that insecurely attached individuals experienced difficulty in trusting and seeking comfort from a partner. This was attributed to the fear of rejection, abandonment, or betrayal that they often lived with due to earlier experiences with attachment figures. The difficulty in establishing trust, coupled with the inability to delay gratification or regulate emotions, posed challenges for establishing healthy, long-lasting relationships, resulting in higher incidence of separation and divorce (Bakermans-Kranenburg & van IJzendoorn, 1997). Attachment anxiety and avoidance impede adaptive coping processes in the aftermath of conflict, and the relational flow of "rupture and repair" is obstructed (Shore, 2003). This increases the risk of emotional problems and maladaptive behaviors, such as evasive behavior or intimate partner violence (Scott & Babcock, 2009; Solomon, Dekel, & Mikulincer, 2008).

A study conducted by Ponti and Tani (2019) found that survivors of domestic violence presented with higher levels of insecurity in their attachment bonds to their mothers and their romantic partners than those who are not abused. This study highlighted a correlation between insecure attachment patterns and intimate partner violence (IPV). The study found that survivors of IPV are more likely to present with avoidant attachment styles toward their partners when compared to not-abused subjects. Other studies have found that perpetration of violence occurs when anxious attachment of perpetrator is in association with the avoidant attachment of the abuse survivor (Pietromonaco, Greenwood, & Feldman Barrett, 2004; Roberts & Noller, 1998). This correlation has been linked to significant differences in two partners' respective need for closeness and differences in their perception of their reciprocal emotional distance. This incongruity is believed to cause hostile communication, denial, aggression, and/or incapacity to provide for the partner's needs (Ponti &

Tani, 2019). A survivor of childhood complex trauma who has used psychotherapy to resolve issues related to shame-based cognition, trust, and vulnerability may see the return of symptoms during major life events, for instance, when adapting to marriage, parenthood, or their own child reaching the age the survivor was when the abuse occurred. The impact of past relational trauma may be awakened at particular points, despite being sufficiently resolved at one stage of recovery in the life cycle (Herman, 1992). Insecure attachment patterns can cause instability and discord in relationships. Consequently, survivors face a higher likelihood of problems in quality of life, social functioning, and emotional well-being.

Attachment Theory Through a Critical Lens

A serious limitation of attachment theory is its failure to recognize the profound influences of social class, gender expression, ethnicity, and culture on personality development. These factors, independent of a caregiver's sensitivity, can be as significant as the quality of the early attachment. Attachment theory's claims and constructs suffer from ethnocentrism; however, relatively few cross-cultural researchers have raised these concerns regarding attachment theory. Within cross-cultural research, the terms race, culture, and ethnicity are often used interchangeably. However, these terms are distinct concepts shaped by political, historical, and socioeconomic norms and practices of a society (Arthur & Collins, 2005). Psychological and anthropological research often regards the Euro-Western (i.e., Caucasian European or American) population as one distinct culture despite the diversity of the heterogeneous group. Cains and Combs-Orme (2005) critique that Euro-Western middle-class families are often considered the norm in comparison with other families. It is unethical to assume that individuals and families of non-Western cultures that resemble this "norm" are superior to their in-group comparisons. Cultural humility must be practiced to honor and respect differences in relation to cultural values.

In White families, the primary attachment figure or caregiver is most often the mother; however, this cultural trend is slowly beginning to change. Conversely within Black communities, there is an Afrocentric value system, which posits that while the biological mother/child bond is valorized, childcare is a collective responsibility (Steele & Steele, 2019). Therefore, caregiving can be viewed as "a situation fostering cooperative, age stratified, woman-centered 'mothering' networks" (Collins, 1987, p. 4). This collective or tribal model of caregiving is not reflected in the design of the Strange Situation experiment. Tomlinson and Swartz (2003) found that the majority of attachment researchers are Euro-Western; therefore, their findings may be impacted by projection, assumption, and cultural bias. Unless researchers are conscientious in their understanding of their own Euro-Western culture and how it influences their behavior and biases, there is a heightened risk of prejudice in their work.

Quinn and Mageo (2013) question the cross-cultural applicability of the category system of attachment theory that designated children's attachment to their caregivers as secure versus insecure. It has been argued that the universality of attachment theory is challenged by a lack of consideration to cultural variation behind the category system and the Strange Situation experimental design. Furthermore, this ethnocentric conceptualization extends beyond the category system into the descriptions of what constitutes an insecure attachment. Attachment takes many forms for people of diverse cultures, ethnicities, and religious groups. Consequentially, misconception of cultural analysis, relationships, connection, and communication can ensue. Rothbaum, Pott, Azuma, Miyake, and Weisz (2000) argue that the assumptions of Euro-Western culture regarding attachment lead Euro-Western researchers to view Japanese caregiving practices as misguided rather than distinctive. For instance, as Japanese caregiving practices inhibit infant exploration, this cultural variation was often pathologized by Euro-Western researchers. Conversely, Guisinger and Blatt (1994) found that Japanese assumptions about attachment perceived Euro-Western relational bonds as being undermined by individualism. The perceived lack of paternal control and uninhibited exploration was viewed as weaker than, rather than distinct from, their own cultural relational values. Opposing cultures often have unique value systems regarding individualism and relatedness (Guisinger & Blatt, 1994; Quinn & Mageo, 2013). Ethnocentric measurements, research, and categorization fail to highlight and valorize the different ways that people around the world conceptualize and engage in close relationships. In short, there are many different ways to develop the parent-child relationship.

Another critique of attachment theory is that it does not account for how the child's temperament and responsivity to the caregiver impacts the bond and the development of epistemic trust. A child who is resistant to attunement and mirroring is at a significant disadvantage in terms of developing a secure attachment to their caregiver. Furthermore, Weber, Levitt, and Clark (1986) suggested that infants may learn avoidant defensive behaviors as a result of oppressive carers who do not attune to the child's inner emerging subjectivity. Infant negative emotionality, that is, an infant's level of distress at limitations, has been found to be strongly correlated with lower quality of bonding (Nolvi et al., 2016). It has also been found that caregivers of irritable infants are more likely to respond in a rigid and controlled manner (Mangelsdorf, Gunnar, Kestenbaum, Lang, & Andreas, 1990; van den Boom, 1989). These findings highlight the role of infant temperament as a contributing factor to early parent-infant relationships and the development of a secure attachment. Further work has indicated that both the caregiver's and the infant's temperament, wider environmental influences, and the caregiver's ability to sensitively attune to the child are key determining factors in the development of attachment pattern (Buss & Plomin, 1984; Goldsmith et al., 1987). Therefore, it is reasoned that the caregiver's sensitivity and the infant's temperament co-create the attachment bond.

Developmental Trauma and Racial Disparity in the Time of COVID-19

A growing body of literature indicates the negative impact of trauma on developmental milestones and brain development, which supports the need to address the prevalence of complex trauma among vulnerable populations (Cloitre, Garvert, Brewin, Bryant, & Maercker, 2013; Hartinger-Saunders, Jones, & Rittner, 2016). Developmental trauma is a term used to describe exposure to trauma in the formative years, which has been found to lead to affective and physiological dysregulation, attentional and behavioral dysregulation, self and relational dysregulation, and post-traumatic stress symptoms (WHO, 2018; van der Kolk et al., 2009). Developmental trauma is associated with complex, layered relational trauma, particularly through childhood abuse and neglect, and has long been recognized in the development of later pathologies.

The spread of the COVID-19 virus has led to many public health challenges, including detrimental mental and physical health outcomes (Fegert, Vitiello, Plener, & Clemens, 2020). In this time of collective trauma, the effects of COVID-19 will undoubtedly give rise to unequal degrees of hardship, primarily impacting those who are most vulnerable to structural and systemic inequality. For instance, Millett et al. (2020) found that US counties with higher populations of Black residents had disproportionately higher rates of COVID-19-related infection and deaths, beyond adjustment for sociodemographics, comorbidities, and socioeconomic determinants. In another study, Azar et al. (2020) found higher rates of COVID-19-related infection among Black adults compared to White patients after adjustment for median household income. Personal and systemic racism and discrimination make accessing healthcare resources very difficult. Kim (2020) argues that disadvantaged communities and people of color experience limited access to health education, hygiene management, and healthy foods. Additionally, they are more likely to reside in densely populated areas and/or live within multigenerational homes, which impedes social distancing, specifically regarding COVID-19. When an individual is in an unequal position in society in terms of stability, security, educational achievements, and employment opportunities, this can be the source of great personal distress (O'Shea Brown, 2020).

Millett et al. (2020) argue that the research findings may underestimate racial/ethnic and socioeconomic disparities as disadvantaged and marginalized groups have less access to primary care physicians. Therefore, the children of minority ethnic groups are far more likely to experience loss, adversity, and hardship due to COVID-19 than their White middle-class peers. On May 25, 2020, Mr. George Floyd, a Black father residing in Minneapolis, was killed in police custody. For 8 minutes and 46 seconds, the arresting officer had his knee pressed on Mr. Floyd's neck, ultimately killing him through asphyxiation. This tragic loss of human life ignited a human rights movement. In the midst of a global pandemic, Mr. Floyd's death further highlighted the racial discrimination and socioeconomic disparities in America. Long before the pandemic, the long-standing epidemics of police brutality and premature death have caused never-ceasing terror for the Black community. In this time of heightened awareness, it is crucial that real and effective change is made to prevent further loss of human life.

As discussed, there is increasing evidence that racial and ethnic minority groups are being disproportionately affected by COVID-19. The long-term psychological impacts of the pandemic, related both to its spread and to the restrictive policies adopted to counteract the spread, remain uncertain. However, recent research has indicated that the precipitous nature of the pandemic along with the widespread uncertainty has the capacity to cause or even exacerbate trauma-related symptoms (Forte, Favieri, Tambelli, & Casagrande, 2020; Shigemura, Ursano, Morganstein, Kurosawa, & Benedek, 2020; Zandifar & Badrfam, 2020). Qualitative data from the countries that were among the first to be impacted has shown an increased rate of anxiety, depression, and PTSD as some of the psychological consequences of the COVID-19 pandemic (Kang et al., 2020; Tan et al., 2020). A systematic review of 13 studies conducted by Pappa et al. (2020) revealed an increased prevalence in the rate of anxiety by 23.2%, depression by 22.8%, and insomnia by 38.9%.

Social distancing, confinement, and quarantine, the steps widely adopted to contain virus transmission, represent drastic changes to normal life (O'Shea Brown, 2021). Together they have altered the fabric of society, creating changes to consciousness and awakening a climate of trepidation. Many individuals struggled to adapt as strong relational bonds, community ties, and the camaraderie and meaning-making provided by education institutes and places of religious practice were abruptly taken away. This abrupt loss of social norms has the potential to activate hypervigilance in many trauma survivors while also creating a large-scale sense of uncertainty characteristic of a global pandemic (Forte et al., 2020). Due to COVID-19's mandated quarantine, there is also decreased access to services that can help mitigate trauma; for instance, as schools close in addition to other community development agencies, children are unlikely to come into contact with mandated reporters organically. This can be detrimental to child welfare as abused or neglected children go under the radar, unseen, and unnoticed. Access to external support by other family members and community-based support systems has also greatly diminished in the wake of COVID-19.

Consequently, circumstantial stress has risen as anxieties related to the pandemic, the economic situation, and overall well-being have proliferated alongside high and rising levels of unemployment in all affected countries (Fegert et al., 2020; Shigemura et al., 2020; Zandifar & Badrfam, 2020). On a societal level, there is a breakdown of trust and an increased level of tension due to the scarcity of resources and support services. Family stressors are also exacerbated. In this time of isolation, dynamics within the dysfunctional family home can be amplified. As proximity magnifies emotions, irritably can develop into rage. There is a heightened risk of domestic violence with more parents and spouses experiencing distress due to employment concerns, health/illness anxiety, and the impacts of isolation (Roesch, Amin, Gupta, & García-Moreno, 2020). These factors can lead to toxic stress and displaced anger, which often results in emotional abuse, physical abuse, and threatening behaviors. When children experience prolonged, repeated interpersonal trauma, this negatively impacts their ability to establish a sense of safety and maintain healthy relationships later in life (Lee & Hankin, 2009; Main & Hesse, 1990; van IJzendoorn, 1995). Experiencing an adverse or traumatic event in childhood predisposes an individual to developing psychopathology, including depression, anxiety, and/or PTSD later on in life (Felitti et al., 1998). The experience of trauma or maltreatment in the formative years creates a vulnerability to severe emotional dysregulation along with intense feelings of despair, anxiety, shame, and mistrust of others later on in life (Wesselmann et al., 2012).

Measuring Attachment Status in a Clinical Setting

Attachment theory and its implications for relationships and overall wellness have led to the development of a variety of assessment methods. Although attachment status has been described by Bowlby as relatively static throughout a lifetime, much research has been conducted to investigate whether adult attachment status can be changed when the insecurely attached individual forges a long-term relationship with a securely attached spouse or engages in long-term psychotherapy (Bakermans-Kranenburg & van IJzendoorn, 1997). Studies of insecurely attached adults found that over 30% of adults demonstrate a change in their attachment pattern from infancy to adulthood, with motivation for positive change identified as an essential catalyst (Davila, Burge, & Hammen, 1997; Kirkpatrick & Hazan, 1994; Ruvolo, Fabin, & Ruvolo, 2001; Scharfe & Bartholomew, 1994; Shaver & Brennan, 1992; Stovall-McClough & Cloitre, 2003; Levy et al., 2006).

There are a number of methods used to measure adult attachment status in a clinical setting, including but not limited to the Adult Attachment Interview (George, Kaplan, & Main, 1985), the Adult Attachment Scale (Hazan & Shaver, 1987), and the Experiences in Close Relationships Questionnaire (Brennan, Clark, & Shaver, 1998). These methods, developed from attachment theory, are a combination of self-reports or interviews. The Adult Attachment Scale (AAS) was officially developed in 1990 but built on the earlier work of Hazan and Shaver (1987) and Levy and Davis (1988). It was designed to classify adults according to the three attachment patterns identified by Ainsworth et al. (1978). The AAS consists of three sets of statements, each describing an attachment pattern (as shown in Box 2.1). An important note is that the Adult Attachment Scale is self-administered; results should be interpreted with the understanding that participants may be answering questions in an aspirational rather than a truthful manner. The AAS assesses the respondent's ability to sustain and tolerate essential relationships in addition to their capacity to trust and be comfortable with vulnerability. The AAS consists of 18 statements scored on a 5-point, Likert-type scale. Adult attachment is measured as "secure," "anxious," and "avoidant." If a respondent scores high in the "close and depend" subscales and low on the anxiety scale, they are deemed to be "secure" in their attachment pattern. If a respondent scores high in the anxiety subscale and low to moderate in "close and depend," they are deemed to be anxious in their attachment pattern. Finally, those who score low on both are deemed to be avoidant in their attachment pattern (see "Scoring Instructions for the Original Adult Attachment Scale" in Box 2.1).

Box 2.1 Adult Attachment Scale (AAS) and Scoring Instructions

Adult Attachment Scale

Please read each of the following statements and rate the extent to which it describes your feelings about romantic relationships. Please think about all your relationships (past and present) and respond in terms of how you generally feel in these relationships. If you have never been involved in a romantic relationship, answer in terms of how you think you would feel.

Please use the scale below by placing a number between 1 and 5 in the space provided to the right of each statement.

1--------------2--------------3--------------4--------------5

Not at all characteristic of me	**Very characteristic of me**

(1) I find it relatively easy to get close to others. ________
(2) I do not worry about being abandoned. ________
(3) I find it difficult to allow myself to depend on others. ________
(4) In relationships, I often worry that my partner does not really love me. ________
(5) I find that others are reluctant to get as close as I would like. ________
(6) I am comfortable depending on others. ________
(7) I do not worry about someone getting too close to me. ________
(8) I find that people are never there when you need them. ________
(9) I am somewhat uncomfortable being close to others. ________
(10) In relationships, I often worry that my partner will not want to stay with me. ________
(11) I want to merge completely with another person. ________
(12) My desire to merge sometimes scares people away. ________
(13) I am comfortable having others depend on me. ________
(14) I know that people will be there when I need them. ________
(15) I am nervous when anyone gets too close. ________
(16) I find it difficult to trust others completely. ________

(continued)

Box 2.1 (continued)

(17) Often, partners want me to be closer than I feel comfortable being. ________

(18) I am not sure that I can always depend on others to be there when I need them. ________

Scoring Instructions for the Original Adult Attachment Scale

The scale contains three subscales, each composed of six items. The three subscales are CLOSE, DEPEND, and ANXIETY. The CLOSE scale measures the extent to which a person is comfortable with closeness and intimacy. The DEPEND scale measures the extent to which a person feels he/she can depend on others to be available when needed. The ANXIETY subscale measures the extent to which a person is worried about being abandoned or unloved.

Original Scoring:

Average the ratings for the six items that compose each subscale as indicated below.

Scale	Items					
CLOSE	1	7	9*	13	15*	17*
DEPEND	3*	6	8*	14	16*	18*
ANXIETY	2*	4	5	10	11	12

* Items with an asterisk should be reverse scored before computing the subscale mean.

Alternative Scoring:

If you would like to compute only *two* attachment dimensions – attachment *anxiety* (model of self) and attachment *avoidance* (model of other) – you can use the following scoring procedure:

Scale	Items											
ANXIETY	2*	4	5	10	11	12						
AVOID	1*	3	6*	7*	8	9	13*	14*	15	16	17	18

* Items with an asterisk should be reverse scored before computing the subscale mean.

Though the Adult Attachment Scale is a useful clinical tool, it is limited in the scope of knowledge we can gather from it in terms of the respondent's relational bonds. Attachment theory postulates that internal working models of attachment are constructed from attachment experiences and that they concern interrelated mental models of self and social life (Bowlby, 1973). The Adult Attachment Interview

(AAI) is used to assess to what extent these experiences were probably characterized by emotional warmth, rejection, neglect, pressure to achieve, or role reversal and, more importantly, the state of mind of the respondent regarding these attachment experiences. The AAI provides a much more personalized and in-depth insight into trust, vulnerability, relational trauma, and the internal working model. It was developed by psychologists Carol George, PhD; Nancy Kaplan, PhD; and Mary Main, PhD, in 1984. It is a quasi-clinical, semi-structured interview that is generally administered by an AAI-trained clinician to the respondent over the duration of 1–2 hours (Cassidy & Shaver, 2008).

The interview involves 20 questions which explore the subject's adult representation of attachment by assessing general and specific recollections from their childhood. The interview is scored based on quality of discourse, especially coherence and content. Categories are designed to ascertain attachment status. It is hypothesized that an adult's evaluation of childhood experiences and their influence on current functioning will become organized into a relatively stable state of mind with regard to attachment (Main, Kaplan, & Cassidy, 1985). The AAI will be explored over the subsequent pages of this chapter; however, please note that this material is not a substitute for training in AAI administration procedure. Seeing the full interview protocol can help consumers of AAI-based research appreciate the intricate levels of interview information and detail underlying AAI scores. For information on training to administer the AAI, please see the Appendix.

Adult Attachment Interview Protocol

Synopsized to Introduction and Questions

Source: George, C., Kaplan, N., & Main, M. (1985). The Adult Attachment Interview. Unpublished manuscript, University of California at Berkeley. Used with permission.

Note: This synopsized overview is for illustration only and not a replacement for training – full information regarding the AAI training is listed in the Appendix.

Introduction

I'm going to be interviewing you about your childhood experiences, and how those experiences may have affected your adult personality. So, I'd like to ask you about your early relationship with your family, and what you think about the way it might have affected you. We'll focus mainly on your childhood, but later we'll get on to your adolescence and then to what's going on right now. This interview often takes about an hour, but it could be anywhere between 45 minutes and an hour and a half.

Questions

- *Could you start by helping me get oriented to your early family situation, and where you lived and so on? If you could tell me where you were born, whether you moved around much, what your family did at various times for a living?*
- *I'd like you to try to describe your relationship with your parents as a young child if you could start from as far back as you can remember?*
  (The intention here is to encourage participants to attempt to remember very early experiences in the formative years).
- *Now I'd like to ask you to choose five adjectives or words that reflect your relationship with your mother, starting from as far back as you can remember in early childhood--as early as you can go, but say, age 5 to 12 is fine. I know this may take a bit of time, so go ahead and think for a minute…then I'd like to ask you why you chose them. I'll write each one down as you give them to me.*
- *Now I'd like to ask you to choose five adjectives or words that reflect your childhood relationship with your father, again starting from as far back as you can remember in early childhood--as early as you can go, but again say, age 5 to 12 is fine. I know this may take a bit of time, so go ahead and think again for a minute…then I'd like to ask you why you chose them. I'll write each one down as you give them to me.*
  (Interviewer repeats with probes as above, it is best to ask these questions in a gender-neutral manner as is LGBTQ affirming for instance 'primary caregiver' and 'other caregiver').
- *Now I wonder if you could tell me, to which parent did you feel the closest, and why? Why isn't there this feeling with the other parent?*
- *When you were upset as a child, what would you do?*
  When you were upset emotionally when you were little, what would you do?
  Can you remember what would happen when you were hurt physically?
  Do any specific incidents come to mind?
- *What is the first time you remember being separated from your parents?*
  How did you respond?
  Do you remember how your parents responded?
  Are there any other separations that stand out in your mind?
- *Did you ever feel rejected as a young child? Of course, looking back on it now, you may realize it wasn't really rejection, but what I'm trying to ask about here is whether you remember ever having felt rejected in childhood.*
- *Were your parents ever threatening with you in any way – maybe for discipline, or even jokingly?*
- *In general, how do you think your overall experiences with your parents have affected your adult personality?*
- *Why do you think your parents behaved as they did during your childhood?*
- *Were there any other adults with whom you were close, like parents, as a child?*
- *Did you experience the loss of a parent or other close loved one while you were a young child--for example, a sibling, or a close family member?*

- *Did you lose any other important persons during your childhood?*
- *Have you lost other close persons, in adult years?*
- *Other than any difficult experiences you've already described, have you had any other experiences which you would regard as potentially traumatic?*
- *Now I'd like to ask you a few more questions about your relationship with your parents. Were there many changes in your relationship with your parents (or remaining parent) after childhood? We'll get to the present in a moment, but right now I mean changes occurring roughly between your childhood and your adulthood?*
- *Now I'd like to ask you, what is your relationship with your parents (or remaining parent) like for you now as an adult? Here I am asking about your current relationship.*
- *If you had three wishes for your child twenty years from now, what would they be? I'm thinking partly of the kind of future you would like to see for your child I'll give you a minute or two to think about this one.*
- *Is there any particular thing which you feel you learned above all from your own childhood experiences?*
- *We've been focusing a lot on the past in this interview, but I'd like to end by looking into the future. We've just talked about what you think you may have learned from your own childhood experiences. I'd like to end by asking you what would you hope your child (or, your imagined child) might have learned from their experiences of being parented by you?*

Summary

Attachment-based clinical work deepens your understanding of an individual's emotional map. It allows you to anticipate challenges and respond appropriately and sensitively. When a client has a secure attachment whereby their childhood needs were adequately met, they can develop trust easily. However, when a childhood is characterized by rejection, humiliation, or neglect, an insecure or disorganized attachment may develop. The insecure attachment can negatively affect their ability to establish a sense of safety and maintain healthy relationships, both personally and in a clinical setting. Vulnerability and the development of trust are especially difficult for the survivor of complex trauma. Thus clinicians working with clients with a history of pervasive relational trauma must be highly conscientious to sensitively attune to and compassionately witness their client. The subsequent chapter shall explore complex layered relational trauma from theoretical and clinical perspectives and consider how it can interfere with an individual's capacity to parent effectively and trust relationally.

Questions and Activities for Discussion and Further Reflection

1. Can you define the following terms: (i) secure attachment, (ii) anxious-insecure, (iii) anxious-avoidant, and (iv) disorganized attachment?
2. What do you see as the social and cultural factors that have the greatest negative impact on attachment?
3. How could attachment theory be evolved and developed to be more inclusive of diverse cultural values and norms?
4. Do you understand attachment as socially constructed?
5. What are the implications of an insecure attachment for parenting, relationships, and the clinical relationship?
6. Identify a client you are working with and think about how you have conceptualized your client up until now. Reflect on how an attachment-informed approach would deepen the work.

Exercise

1. Class Discussion Prompt: Reflect on the narrative of your formative years and life experience today. How has this shaped and informed your attachment patterns? Do you believe insecure attachment is an injury or a disorder?
2. Self-administer the Adult Attachment Scale – Any personal reflections on the questionnaire are welcome in a smaller group discussion (3–5 students per group).
3. Assignment Suggestion: Choose one question from the AAI and answer it as thoughtfully and in as much depth as you can.

References

Ainsworth, M. D. S. (1967). *Infancy in Uganda: Infant care and the growth of love*. Baltimore, MD: Johns Hopkins University Press.
Ainsworth, M. D. S. (1982). Attachment: Retrospect and prospect. In C. M. Parkes & J. Stevenson-Hinde (Eds.), *The place of attachment in human behavior* (pp. 3–29). New York, NY: Tavistock.
Ainsworth, M. D. S., & Bell, S. M. (1970). Attachment, exploration, and separation: Illustrated by the behavior of one-year-olds in a strange situation. *Child Development, 41*, 49–67.
Ainsworth, M. D. S., Blehar, M. C., Waters, E., & Wall, S. (1978). *Patterns of attachment: A psychological study of the strange situation*. Hillsdale, NJ: Lawrence Erlbaum.
American Psychiatric Association. (2013). *Diagnostic and statistical manual of mental disorders* (5th ed.). Washington, DC: American Psychiatric Publishing.
Arthur, N., & Collins, S. (2005). Introduction to culture-infused counselling. In N. Arthur & S. Collins (Eds.), *Culture-infused counselling: Celebrating the Canadian mosaic*. Counselling Concepts: Calgary, AB.
Azar, K. M. J., Shen, Z., Romanelli, R. J., Lockhart, S. H., Smits, K., & Robinson, S. (2020). Disparities in outcomes among COVID-19 patients in a large health care system in California. *Health Affairs (Millwood), 39*, 1253–1262.

Bakermans-Kranenburg, M. J., & van IJzendoorn, M. H. (1997). Adult attachment and the break-up of romantic relationships. *Journal of Divorce and Remarriage, 27*, 121–139.
Bowlby, J. (1969/1982). *Attachment and loss: Vol. 1. Attachment*. New York, NY: Basic Books.
Bowlby, J. (1973). *Separation: Anxiety and anger* (Psychology of attachment and loss series) (Vol. 3). New York, NY: Basic Books.
Bowlby, J. (1980). *Attachment and loss, III: Loss, sadness, and depression*. New York, NY: Basic Books.
Bowlby, J. (1989). The role of attachment in personality development and psychopathology. In S. I. Greenspan & G. H. Pollack (Eds.), *The course of life: Vol. 1. Infancy* (pp. 119–136). Madison, CT: International Universities Press.
Brennan, K. A., Clark, C. L., & Shaver, P. R. (1998). Self-report measurement of adult attachment: An integrative overview. In J. A. Simpson & W. S. Rholes (Eds.), *Attachment theory and close relationships* (pp. 46–76). New York, NY: Guilford Press.
Buss, A., & Plomin, R. (1984). *Temperament: Early developing personality traits*. Hillsdale, NJ: Lawrence Erlbaum Associates.
Cains, D. S., & Combs-Orme, T. (2005). Family structure effects on parenting stress and practices in the African American family. *Journal of Sociology and Social Welfare, 32*(2), 19–40.
Carlson, E. A. (1998). A prospective longitudinal study of attachment disorganization/disorientation. *Child Development, 69*(4), 1107–1128.
Cassidy, J., & Shaver, P. (Eds.). (2008). *Handbook of attachment: Theory, research, and clinical applications* (2nd ed.). The Guilford Press.
Chartrand, T. L., & Bargh, J. (1999). The chameleon effect: The perception-behavior link and social interaction. *Journal of Personality and Social Psychology, 76*, 893–910.
Cloitre, M., Garvert, D. W., Brewin, C. R., Bryant, R. A., & Maercker, A. (2013). Evidence for proposed ICD-11 PTSD and complex PTSD: A latent profile analysis. *European Journal of Psychotraumatology, 4*, 20706. https://doi.org/10.3402/ejpt.v4i0.20706
Collins, N. L., & Read, S. J. (1990). Adult attachment, working models, and relationship quality in dating couples. *Journal of Personality and Social Psychology, 58*, 644–663.
Collins, P. H. (1987). The meaning of motherhood in black culture and black mother/daughter relationships. *SAGE: A Scholarly Journal on Black Women, 4*(2), 3–10.
Corriveau, K. H., Harris, P. L., Meins, E., Fernyhough, C., Arnott, B., Elliott, L., & de Rosnay, M. (2009). Young children's trust in their mother's claims: Longitudinal links with attachment security in infancy. *Child Development, 80*, 750–761.
Davila, J., Burge, D., & Hammen, C. (1997). Why does attachment change? *Journal of Personality and Social Psychology, 73*(4), 826–838.
De Wolff, M., & van IJzendoorn, M. H. (1997). Sensitivity and attachment: A meta-analysis on parental antecedents of infant attachment. *Child Development, 68*(4), 571–591. https://doi.org/10.2307/1132107
Fegert, J., Vitiello, B., Plener, P. L., & Clemens, V. (2020). Challenges and burden of the coronavirus 2019 (COVID-19) pandemic for child and adolescent mental health: A narrative review to highlight clinical and research needs in the acute phase and the long return to normality. *Child and Adolescent Psychiatry and Mental Health, 14*, 1–11. http://dx.doi.org.proxy.library.nyu.edu/10.1186/s13034-020-00329-3
Felitti, V. J., Anda, R. F., Nordenberg, D., Williamson, D. F., Spitz, A. M., Edwards, V., … Marks, J. S. (1998). Relationship of childhood abuse and household dysfunction to many of the leading causes of death in adults. The adverse childhood experiences (ACE) study. *American Journal of Preventive Medicine, 14*, 245–258.
Fonagy, P., Gergely, G., & Target, M. (2007). The parent-infant dyad and the construction of the subjective self. *Journal of Child Psychology and Psychiatry, 48*, 288–328. https://doi.org/10.1111/j.1469-7610.2007.01727.x
Forte, G., Favieri, F., Tambelli, R., & Casagrande, M. (2020). COVID-19 pandemic in the Italian population: Validation of a post-traumatic stress disorder questionnaire and prevalence of

PTSD symptomatology. *International Journal of Environmental Research and Public Health, 17*(11), 4151. http://dx.doi.org.proxy.library.nyu.edu/10.3390/ijerph17114151

George, C., Kaplan, N., & Main, M. (1985). *The adult attachment interview*. Unpublished manuscript, University of California at Berkeley.

George, C., & Solomon, J. (2011). *Disorganized attachment and caregiving*. New York, NY: Guilford Press.

Goldsmith, H. H., Buss, A. H., Plomin, R., Rothbart, M. K., Thomas, A., Chess, S., … McCall, R. B. (1987). Roundtable: What is temperament? Four approaches. *Child Development, 58*, 505–529.

Granqvist, P., Sroufe, L. A., Dozier, M., Hesse, E., Steele, M., Van IJzendoorn, M., & Duschinsky, R. (2017). Disorganized attachment in infancy: A review of the phenomenon and its implications for clinicians and policy-makers. *Attachment & Human Development, 19*(6), 534–558. https://doi.org/10.1080/14616734.2017.1354040

Grossmann, K., Fremmer-Bombik, E., Rudolph, J., & Grossmann, K. E. (1988). Maternal attachment representations as related to patterns of infant-mother attachment and maternal care during the first year. In R. A. Hinde & J. Stevenson-Hinde (Eds.), *Relationships within families: Mutual influences* (pp. 241–260). Oxford, UK: Clarendon Press.

Guisinger, S., & Blatt, S. J. (1994). Individuality and relatedness: Evolution of a fundamental dialectic. *American Psychologist, 49*, 104–111.

Hartinger-Saunders, R. M., Jones, A. S., & Rittner, B. (2016). Improving access to trauma-informed adoption services: Applying a developmental trauma framework. *Journal of Child & Adolescent Trauma, 12*(1), 119–130. https://doi.org/10.1007/s40653-016-0104-1

Hazan, C., & Shaver, P. (1987). Romantic love conceptualized as an attachment process. *Journal of Personality and Social Psychology., 52*, 511–524.

Herman, J. L. (1992). *Trauma and recovery: The aftermath of violence*. New York, NY: Basic Books.

Hertsgaard, L., Gunnar, M., Erickson, M. F., & Nachmias, M. (1995). Adrenocortical responses to the strange situation in infants with disorganized/disoriented attachment relationships. *Child Development, 66*, 1100–1106.

Kang, L., Ma, S., Chen, M., Yang, J., Wang, Y., Li, R., … Liu, Z. (2020). Impact on mental health and perceptions of psychological care among medical and nursing staff in Wuhan during the 2019 novel coronavirus disease outbreak: A cross-sectional study. *Brain, Behavior, and Immunity, 87*, 11–17. https://doi.org/10.1016/j.bbi.2020.03.028

Kim, J. (2020). Equality, inclusion, and diversity in healthcare during the COVID-19 pandemic. *International Neurourology Journal, 24*, 180–181.

Kirkpatrick, L. A., & Hazan, C. (1994). Attachment styles and close relationships: A four–year prospective study. *Personal Relationships, 1*, 123–142.

Lee, A., & Hankin, B. L. (2009). Insecure attachment, dysfunctional attitudes, and low self-esteem predicting prospective symptoms of depression and anxiety during adolescence. *Journal of Clinical Child and Adolescent Psychology: The Official Journal for the Society of Clinical Child and Adolescent Psychology, American Psychological Association, 38*(2), 219–231.

Levy, M. B., & Davis, K. E. (1988). Lovestyles and Attachment Styles Compared: Their Relations to Each Other and to Various Relationship Characteristics. *Journal of Social and Personal Relationships, 5*(4), 439–471. https://doi.org/10.1177/0265407588054004

Levy, K. N., Meehan, K. B., Kelly, K. M., Reynoso, J. S., Weber, M., Clarkin, J. F., et al. (2006). Change in attachment and reflective function in the treatment of borderline personality disorder with transference focused psychotherapy. *Journal of Consulting and Clinical Psychology, 74*, 1027–1040.

Lyons-Ruth, K., & Jacobvitz, D. (2008). Attachment disorganization: Genetic factors, parenting contexts, and developmental transformation from infancy to adulthood. In *Handbook of attachment: Theory, research, and clinical applications* (2nd ed., pp. 666–697). New York, NY: Guilford Press.

Main, M., & Cassidy, J. (1988). Categories of response to reunion with the parent at age 6: Predictable from infant attachment classifications and stable over a 1-month period. *Developmental Psychology, 24*, 415–426.

Main, M., & Hesse, E. (1990). Parents' unresolved traumatic experiences are related to infant disorganized attachment status: Is frightened and/or frightening parental behavior the linking mechanism? In M. Greenberg, D. Cichetti, & M. Cummings (Eds.), *Attachment in the preschool years* (pp. 161–182). Chicago, IL: University of Chicago Press, Division 53, 38(2), pp. 219–231. https://doi.org/10.1080/15374410802698396

Main, M., Kaplan, N., & Cassidy, J. (1985). Security in infancy, childhood, and adulthood: A move to the level of representation. *Monographs of the Society for Research in Child Development, 50*(1–2), 66–104. https://doi.org/10.2307/3333827

Main, M., & Solomon, J. (1986). Discovery of an insecure-disorganized/disoriented attachment pattern. In T. B. Brazelton & M. Yogman (Eds.), *Affective development in infancy* (pp. 95–124). Norwood, NJ: Ablex.

Main, M., & Solomon, J. (1990). Procedures for identifying infants as disorganized/disoriented during the Ainsworth Strange Situation. In *Attachment in the preschool years: Theory, research, and intervention* (pp. 121–160). Chicago, IL: University of Chicago Press.

Mangelsdorf, S. C., Gunnar, M., Kestenbaum, R., Lang, S., & Andreas, D. (1990). Infant proneness-to-distress temperament, maternal personality, and mother-infant attachment: Associations and the goodness of fit. *Child Development, 61*, 820–831.

Millett, G. A., Jones, A. T., Benkeser, D., Baral, S., Mercer, L., Beyrer, C., … Sullivan, P. (2020). Assessing differential impacts of COVID-19 on black communities. *Annals of Epidemiology, 47*, 37–44.

Mischel, W. (2014). *The marshmallow test – Why self-control is the engine of success*. New York, NY: Little, Brown & Co.

Mischel, W., Ayduk, O., Berman, M. G., Casey, B. J., Gotlib, I. H., Jonides, J., … Shoda, Y. (2011). "Willpower" over the 107 life span: Decomposing self-regulation. *Social Cognitive and Affective Neuroscience, 6*(2), 252–256. https://doi.org/10.1093/scan/nsq081

NICHD. (1998). Early child care and self-control, compliance, and problem behavior at twenty-four and thirty-six months. *Child Development, 69*(4), 1145. https://doi.org/10.2307/1132367

Nolvi, S., Karlsson, L., Bridgett, D. J., Pajulo, M., Tolvanen, M., & Karlsson, H. (2016). Maternal postnatal psychiatric symptoms and infant temperament affect early mother-infant bonding. *Infant Behavior & Development, 43*, 13–23. pmid:27054496

O'Shea Brown, G. (2020). The impact of anomie and societal splitting on the self: Suicide among members of the travelling Community of Ireland. *Journal of PsychoHistory, 48*(2).

O'Shea Brown, G. (2021). Reflections on providing virtual eye movement desensitization and reprocessing therapy in the wake of COVID-19: Survival through adaptation. In C. Tosone (Ed.), *Shared trauma, shared resilience during a pandemic: Social work in the time of COVID-19*. Cham, Switzerland: Springer.

Pappa, S., Ntella, V., Giannakas, T., Giannakoulis, V. G., Papoutsi, E., & Katsaounou, P. (2020). Prevalence of depression, anxiety, and insomnia among healthcare workers during the COVID-19 pandemic: A systematic review and meta-analysis. *Brain, Behavior, and Immunity*. https://doi.org/10.1016/j.bbi.2020.05.026.

Pietromonaco, P. R., Greenwood, D., & Feldman Barrett, L. (2004). Conflict in adult close relationships: An attachment perspective. In W. S. Rholes & J. A. Simpson (Eds.), *Adult attachment: New directions and emerging issues* (pp. 267–299). New York, NY: Guilford Press.

Ponti, L., & Tani, F. (2019). Attachment bonds as risk factors of intimate partner violence. *Journal of Child and Family Studies, 28*(5), 1425–1432. http://dx.doi.org.proxy.library.nyu.edu/10.1007/s10826-019-01361-4

Quinn, N., & Mageo, J. M. (2013). Attachment and culture: An introduction. In N. Quinn & J. M. Mageo (Eds.), *Attachment reconsidered. Culture, mind, and society* (The book series of the society for psychological anthropology). New York, NY: Palgrave Macmillan. https://doi.org/10.1057/9781137386724_1

Roberts, N., & Noller, P. (1998). The associations between adult attachment and couple violence: The role of communication patterns and relationship satisfaction. In J. A. Simpson & W. S. Rholes (Eds.), *Attachment theory and close relationships* (pp. 317–350). New York, NY: Guilford Press.

Roesch, E., Amin, A., Gupta, J., & García-Moreno, C. (2020). Violence against women during COVID-19 pandemic restrictions. *BMJ: British Medical Journal (Online), 369*. http://dx.doi.org.proxy.library.nyu.edu/10.1136/bmj.m1712

Rothbaum, F., Pott, M., Azuma, H., Miyake, K., & Weisz, J. (2000). The development of close relationships in Japan and the United States: Paths of symbiotic harmony and generative tension. *Child Development, 71*(5), 1121–1142. https://doi.org/10.1111/1467-8624.00214

Ruvolo, A. P., Fabin, L. A., & Ruvolo, C. M. (2001). Relationship experiences and change in attachment characteristics of young adults: The role of relationship breakups and conflict avoidance. *Personal Relationships, 8*, 265–281.

Scharfe, E., & Bartholomew, K. (1994). Reliability and stability of adult attachment patterns. *Personal Relationships, 1*, 23–44.

Scott, S., & Babcock, J. C. (2009). Attachment as a moderator between intimate partner violence and PTSD symptoms. *Journal of Family Violence, 25*(1), 1–9. https://doi.org/10.1007/s10896-009-pp.9264-1

Shaver, P. R., & Brennan, K. A. (1992). Attachment styles and the "Big Five" personality traits: Their connections with each other and with romantic relationship outcomes. *Personality and Social Psychology Bulletin, 18*(5), 536–545. https://doi.org/10.1177/0146167292185003.

Shigemura, J., Ursano, R. J., Morganstein, J. C., Kurosawa, M., & Benedek D. M. (2020). Public responses to the novel 2019 coronavirus (2019 – nCoV): Mental health consequences and target populations. Psychiatry and Clinical Neurosciences. [Epub ahead of print].

Shore, A. (2003). *Affect dysregulation and disorders of the self*. New York, NY: Norton.

Solomon, J., George, C., & De Jong, A. (1995). Children classified as controlling at age six: Evidence of disorganized representational strategies and aggression at home and at school. *Development and Psychopathology, 7*, 447–463.

Solomon, Z., Dekel, R., & Mikulincer, M. (2008). Complex trauma of war captivity: A prospective study of attachment and post-traumatic stress disorder. *Psychological Medicine, 38*, 1427–1434.

Steele, M., & Steele, P. (2019). *Handbook of attachment based interventions*. New York, NY: Guilford Press.

Stovall-McClough, K. C., & Cloitre, M. (2003). Reorganization of unresolved childhood traumatic memories following exposure therapy. *Annals of the New York Academy of Sciences, 1008*, 297–299. https://doi.org/10.1196/annals.1301.036

Tan, B. Y. Q., Chew, N. W. S., Lee, G. K. H., Jing, M., Goh, Y., Yeo, L. L. L., Zhang, K., Chin, H.-K., Ahmad, A., Khan, F. A., Shanmugam, G. N., Chan, B. P. L., Sunny, S., Chandra, B., Ong, J. J. Y., Paliwal, P. R., Wong, L. Y. H., Sagayanathan … Sharma, V. K. (2020). Psychological impact of the COVID-19 pandemic on 2 9 health care workers in Singapore. *Annals of Internal Medicine, 173*(4), 317–320. https://doi.org/10.7326/M20-1083

Tomlinson, M., & Swartz, L. (2003). Imbalances in the knowledge about infancy: The divide between rich and poor countries. *Infant Mental Health Journal, 24*(6), 547–556.

Tronick, E., Als, H., Adamson, L., Wise, S., & Brazelton, T. B. (1978). The infant's response to entrapment between contradictory messages in face-to-face interaction. *Journal of the American Academy of Child and Adolescent Psychiatry, 17*, 1–13.

Tronick, E., & Gold, C. (2020). *The power of discord: Why ups and downs of relationships are the secret to building intimacy, resilience, and trust*. New York, NY: Hachette Book Club.

van den Boom, D. C. (1989). Irritability as an aspect of temperament. In G. A. Kohnstamm, J. E. Bates, & M. K. Rothbart (Eds.), *Temperament in childhood*. New York, NY: Wiley.

van der Kolk, B., Pynoos, R., Cicchetti, D., Cloitre, M., D'Andrea, W., Ford, J., & Teicher, M. (2009). *Proposal to include a developmental trauma disorder diagnosis for children and adolescents in DSM-V*. Available online at http://www.traumacenter.org/announcements/dtd_papers_oct_09.pdf

van IJzendoorn, M. H. (1992). Intergenerational transmission of parenting: A review of studies in nonclinical populations. *Developmental Review, 12*, 76–99.
van IJzendoorn, M. H. (1995). Adult attachment representations, parental responsiveness, and infant attachment: A meta-analysis on the predictive validity of the adult attachment interview. *Psychological Bulletin, 117*, 387–403.
Weber, R. A., Levitt, M. J., & Clark, M. C. (1986). Individual verification in attachment security and strange situation behavior: The role of maternal and infant temperament. *Child Development, 57*, 56–65.
Wesselmann, D. (2013, April). *Using EMDR to treat attachment trauma in adults and children*. Preconference presentation at the Congress EMDR Vereniging EMDR Nederland, The Netherlands, Nijmegen.
Wesselmann, D., Davidson, M., Armstrong, S., Schweitzer, C., Bruckner, D., & Potter, A. E. (2012). EMDR as a treatment for improving attachment status in adults and children. *European Review of Applied Psychology, 62*, 223–230.
World Health Organization [WHO]. (2018). *The ICD-11 for mortality and morbidity statistics*. Retrieved from https://icd-who-int.proxy.library.nyu.edu/browse11/l-m/en
Zandifar, A., & Badrfam, R. (2020). Iranian mental health during the COVID-19 epidemic. *Asian Journal of Psychiatry., 51*, 10199.

Chapter 3
Complex Layered Trauma

Trauma informs identity not just through the development of maladaptive behaviors such as hypervigilance and psychological reactivity to events but also through the formation of shame-based cognition (Herman, 1992; Shapiro & Forrest, 2016). The following quote from Shakespeare's *Henry IV* depicts a concerned wife's observations of her husband's symptoms of posttraumatic stress as he anticipates returning to the trauma of the battlefield. She speaks of his night terrors, flashbacks, and pervasive shame-based cognition derived from survivor's guilt:

> *... my good lord, why are you thus alone? [...] Why dost thou bend thine eyes upon the earth, and start so often when thou sit'st alone? [...] In thy faint slumbers, I by thee have watched, and heard thee murmur tales of iron war [...] thou hast talk'd, of sallies and retires, of trenches, tents [...] Of prisoners' ransom and of soldiers slain, and all the currents of a heady fight. Thy spirit within thee hath been so at war, and thus hath so bestirred thee in thy sleep, that beads of sweat have stood upon thy brow like bubbles in a late-disturbed stream.* (Shakespeare, 1564–1616)

While posttraumatic stress has been recognized in the works of Shakespeare, Homer, and other great historical writers, psychiatry did not fully recognize its existence until 1980 when posttraumatic stress disorder (PTSD) was introduced into the *Diagnostic and Statistical Manual of Mental Disorders, Third Edition* (DSM-III) (American Psychiatric Association, 1980).

English physician Charles Myers, who wrote the first paper on "shell shock," posited that its symptoms stemmed from a physical injury. Myers (1916) theorized that when veterans experienced repeated exposure to concussive blasts, this caused brain trauma that resulted in a strange grouping of symptoms known as "shell shock." Symptoms included but were not limited to alcoholism, substance abuse, mood disorder, hypervigilance, flashbacks, and even schizophrenia. However, when Myers' hypothesis was tested, it was invalidated, as even veterans who had not endured direct physical trauma from the battlefield exhibited symptoms of "shell shock" (Jones, 2010). It was not until 1980 when a group of Vietnam veterans eventually aided New York psychoanalysts Chaim Shatan and Robert J. Lifton in

G. O'Shea Brown, *Healing Complex Posttraumatic Stress Disorder*, Essential Clinical Social Work Series, https://doi.org/10.1007/978-3-030-61416-4_3

successfully lobbying the American Psychiatric Association (APA) to create a new diagnosis identifying what had been called "shell shock" as a specific psychological syndrome (Grant, 2020). PTSD detailed symptoms that were common to most but not all veterans; this created a conceptual framework which set the stage for radical change and reformation in trauma-informed care and research (van der Kolk, 2015).

The *Diagnostic and Statistical Manual of Mental Disorders* (DSM) places the symptoms of PTSD into four main areas: (1) recurrent experiencing of the traumatic event through nightmares, intrusive images, and physiological reactivity to reminders of the trauma; (2) avoidance of thoughts, feelings, or reminders of the trauma; (3) negative cognition and mood; and (4) arousal and reactivity in the form of hypervigilance and an exaggerated startle response (American Psychological Association, 2013). These symptoms have been shown to inhibit the trauma survivor's capacity to establish trust, tolerate stabilization, and navigate a core sense of self. PTSD manifests differently in individuals in terms of severity, chronicity, and impact on quality of life. Financial hardship and a lack of social support have been cited as risk factors in the development of PTSD (APA, 2013). The DSM does not conceptualize PTSD as a normal response to an abnormal behavior. Rather, it views PTSD as a pathological response to an extreme form of stress stored in the memory, for instance, following the death of a loved one or a diagnosis of chronic illness or in the aftermath of an assault (McNally, 2006).

Acute stress disorder (ASD) is a diagnosis given from 3 days to 1 month following a traumatic event, commonly referred to as the acute phase (APA, 2013). If posttraumatic stress symptoms persist beyond a month, the clinician would assess for the presence of PTSD (see subsection "Measuring Trauma in a Clinical Setting"). The ASD diagnosis would no longer apply, and, controversially, the diagnosis of PTSD is indicative of a pathological or prolonged response to the trauma. This has been seen as controversial as it places a very definite timeframe on what is deemed an acceptable grieving or rebounding period after a trauma or loss. It has been suggested that this strict timeframe does not allow for flexibility in understanding an individual's unique circumstances or the nature of the traumatic stress. A diagnosis of ASD has proven beneficial in facilitating access to healthcare after trauma exposure. However, a debate continues regarding ASD as a predictor of posttraumatic stress disorder. Furthermore, it must be noted that ASD does not account for non-fear-based symptoms and/or dissociation, which would fall under the category of PTSD (discussed further in Chaps. 5 and 6).

The diagnostic symptom criteria of PTSD include non-fear-based symptoms, such as risky or destructive behavior; overly negative self-concept; exaggerated blame of self or others for causing the trauma; negative affect; decreased interest in activities; and feelings of isolation (APA, 2013). Furthermore, dissociative symptoms such as depersonalization and derealization are included as symptoms under PTSD but not ASD (see more on dissociative categories in Chap. 5). A diagnosis of PTSD has been helpful in understanding and treating single incident trauma, including trauma resulting from a rape, a physical assault, or traumatic experiences during war. However, the impact of prolonged interpersonal traumatization beginning in childhood was generally overlooked in the early years following the creation of the

PTSD diagnosis. Over time, the term "complex trauma" began to be used to describe chronic traumatization, for instance, the experience of multiple and/or prolonged developmentally adverse traumatic events, most often of an interpersonal nature (Herman, 1992).

This chapter will first provide an exploration of the emergence of complex posttraumatic stress disorder (C-PTSD) with an overview of symptoms and an explanation of how C-PTSD is unique from other diagnoses. Secondly, this chapter examines insecure attachment and relational trauma as diathetic factors to the development of C-PTSD. Following this overview, the neuroscience of complex trauma with specific attention to the mind-body connection will be critically explored. Subsequently, this chapter will present interventions utilized to measure the impact of trauma in a clinical setting.

Emergence of C-PTSD

In 1992, Herman proposed C-PTSD as a unique clinical syndrome following precipitating traumatic events that are prolonged and of an interpersonal nature. C-PTSD denotes a severe form of PTSD and is the result of chronic, prolonged, and repeated trauma arising from childhood abuse, neglect, and/or exposure to domestic violence. C-PTSD is associated with a broad spectrum of psychopathological symptoms and transcends the category of posttraumatic stress disorder (Herman, 1992). C-PTSD is conceptualized as including the core elements of PTSD, such as re-experiencing, avoidance, and hypervigilance, with additional symptoms of poor affect regulation, negative self-concept, and difficulties with establishing and maintaining healthy interpersonal relationships (van der Kolk, 2015; Cloitre et al., 2011; van der van der Kolk, Roth, Pelcovitz, Sunday, & Spinazzola, 2005). The recognition of C-PTSD, its root causes, and its impact demonstrates that childhood trauma, including abuse and neglect, is a major public health concern. Yet the challenge it poses has the potential to be largely resolved by appropriate prevention and intervention.

Complex trauma is the result of chronic, prolonged, and repeated trauma arising from childhood abuse, neglect, and/or exposure to domestic violence. The work of Judith Herman MD (1992) highlighted how survivors of complex relational trauma often present as consumed with shame, distrustful, and actively wounded years or even decades after their so-called escape to freedom. "Many abused children cling to the hope that growing up will bring escape and freedom…But the personality formed in the environment of coercive control is not well adapted to adult life. The survivor is left with fundamental problems in basic trust, autonomy, and initiative… (As an adult, the survivor is) burdened by major impairments in self-care, in cognition and in memory, in identity, and in the capacity to form stable relationships. (They remain) a prisoner of (their) childhood; attempting to create a new life, (but still) reencountering the trauma" (Herman, 1992, p. 80). Herman (1992) began to shine a light on the pain endured by survivors of complex trauma. An insidious aspect of complex trauma is that it usually begins in the home, and a vast majority of those responsible for child maltreatment are the children's own parent(s) (Felitti et al., 1998). Inquiry into developmental milestones and family medical history is routine in medical and psychiatric examinations; however, it is concerning that obtaining information about childhood trauma, abuse, neglect, and other exposures to violence is not (van der Kolk, 2005).

Research has found that adult survivors of clustered adverse childhood experiences go on to develop high-risk maladaptive behaviors, difficulty in establishing and maintaining healthy relationships, mental distress, and poor physical health (Felitti et al., 1998; Centers for Disease Control and Prevention, 2014). Poignantly, the adverse childhood experiences (ACE) study also identified that survivors are at an increased risk for suicidality and overall impulsivity. Among survivors of childhood trauma, an impulse to ritualistically and compulsively seek comfort is common and leads to a higher prevalence of addiction. Chronic traumatization in the formative years has been linked to depression, various medical illnesses, and a variety of impulsive, self-destructive behaviors (van der Kolk, 2005; van der van der Kolk et al., 2005). The DSM IV Field Trial (van der Kolk, McFarlane, & Weisaeth, 1996) petitioned to have complex posttraumatic disorder entered as a unique diagnosis, reasoning that chronic traumatization and the experience of multiple and/or chronic prolonged, developmentally adverse traumatic events were not adequately characterized by PTSD. The DSM IV Field Trial demonstrated that it was not the prevalence of PTSD symptoms themselves but depression, outbursts of anger, shame, distrust for others, and self-destructive or risky behaviors that distinguished C-PTSD from PTSD.

Developing a new psychiatric diagnosis requires that it be validated as a distinct entity with a clinical utility (APA, 2013). Some mental health professionals argued that C-PTSD overlapped in symptomology with several mental disorders following trauma, mainly PTSD, which is usually correlated to single event trauma, as well as borderline personality disorder (BPD). BPD is often comorbid with C-PTSD and shares some of the core symptoms such as impaired relationships with others, dissociative symptoms, impulsive or reckless behaviors, irritability, and the presence self-destructive behaviors. However, C-PTSD is defined by symptom clusters mainly resembling an enhanced PTSD, with symptoms such as shame-based cognition, hypervigilance, social withdrawal, despair, and somatization. Consequently, C-PTSD differs significantly from BPD (Giourou et al., 2018). C-PTSD was under consideration to be included in the DSM-4 (1994) and again in DSM-5 (2013), but was excluded on both occasions for reasons of symptom overlap. However, the following addition was placed in the introductory paragraph to the trauma- and stressor-related disorders section of DSM-5: "It is clear, however, that many individuals who have been exposed to a traumatic or stressful event exhibit a phenotype in which, rather than anxiety- or fear-based symptoms, the most prominent clinical characteristics are anhedonic and dysphoric symptoms, externalizing angry and aggressive symptoms, or dissociative symptoms" (APA, 2013). This addition to the DSM-5 is helpful to clinicians in understanding, diagnosing, and treating some aspects of C-PTSD. However, affect dysregulation, dissociation, and negative self-concept arising from relational and developmental trauma simply are not captured with the classic PTSD diagnostic criteria. Alas, a gap in guidance for diagnosing, treating, and healing complex trauma has become increasingly more evident.

Deconstructing C-PTSD: A Diathesis-Stress Model Perspective

The negative effects of layered relational trauma, particularly as experienced through childhood abuse and neglect, have long been recognized as contributing factors toward the development of C-PTSD (Courtois, 1988; van der Kolk, 2015), a diagnostic entity included in the *International Classification of Diseases, 11th revision* (*ICD-11*). According to the *ICD-11*, C-PTSD is associated with a broad spectrum of psychopathological symptoms and is conceptualized as including the core elements of PTSD such as re-experiencing the trauma, deliberate avoidance of internal and external traumatic reminders, and a sense of current threat expressed as hypervigilance and hyperarousal. The *ICD-11* has also recently identified additional C-PTSD symptoms, including emotional regulation difficulties, persistent negative views of the self, and interpersonal problems characterized by difficulties forming and maintaining relationships with others (WHO, 2018). Until recently, C-PTSD was never officially codified in any diagnostic nomenclature. Endorsement of the *ICD-11* definition of C-PTSD will come into effect on January 1, 2022.

Trauma informs identity not just through the development of maladaptive behaviors, such as hypervigilance and psychological reactivity to events, but also through the formation of shame-based cognition (Shapiro, 2014; Shapiro & Forrest, 2016). Many children will adopt a moral defense as a coping strategy, blaming themselves for their parent's ineffective parenting. Fairbairn (1943) originated "the Moral Defense Against Bad Objects," explaining that it was a defensive strategy applied by children to lessen their anxiety about being dependent on objects who continuously frustrated their needs. The children Dr. Fairbairn studied were obviously neglected and came from abusive families; however, they vehemently defended their parents when he questioned them about the abuse. He was astonished by how eager the abused children were to blame themselves for the neglect and/or abuse. They internalized the "badness" of their parental objects as a defensive strategy. Children have such limited control and agency in their lives that they adopt the moral defense in an attempt to assume a heightened sense of control and responsibility, even for traumatic events (O'Shea Brown, 2020). Although traumatic events in the formative years are incidents which the child simply has no control over, the child will internalize his, her, or their central negative belief (O'Shea Brown, 2020). This is what leads to the development of shame-based cognition.

A diathesis-stress model is a psychological model that frames a disorder in terms of a hereditary disposition (diathesis) interacting with negative life experiences (stressors). A diathesis-stress model posits that when an individual experiences adverse life events in the formative years, one develops a negative self-schema (Slavich & Auerbach, 2018). This schema remains dormant until an individual experiences a traumatic life event that is reminiscent of the original stressor, at which point the preexisting schema or vulnerability becomes activated as a central negative cognition (Slavich & Auerbach, 2018). Experiencing an adverse or traumatic event in one's childhood predisposes the individual to developing a psychopathology such as C-PTSD later on in life (van der Kolk, 2015). According to the additive model, an individual with a significant diathesis may only require a minor stressor or adverse life experience for a disorder to develop (Rutter, 2007). Maltreatment by parents is a direct precursor to the development of disorganized attachment in children, with the majority of maltreated children experiencing difficulty in trusting and seeking comfort in relationships (Granqvist et al., 2017). Collins and Read (1990) attributed this to the fear of rejection, abandonment, or betrayal that they often lived with due to earlier experiences with attachment figures. The psychological phenomenon of one's inclination to reenact traumatic events and their circumstances has been coined as "repetition compulsion" (Freud, 1914). Repetition compulsion is attributed to our predisposition to feel comfortable in the familiar in addition to experiencing the desire to return to an earlier state of things. Returning back to the familiar can be driven by a desire to rewrite the past. Unconsciously drifting to the familiar is driven by a reparation fantasy, a desire to rewrite the past and thus triumph over the pain experienced at an earlier time (Freud, 1914). This desire creates a mirage that one can master the sensation of pain and loss. However, repetition compulsion can cause retraumatization and further shame for the trauma survivor. This repeated pattern of relational trauma reenactment has been referred to as "the bite that fits the wound" (Takin & Hendrix, 2011). The current activation of old attachment wounds can be both familiar and deeply painful.

The case of Monique[1] illustrates how a 36-year-old divorced black female survivor of domestic violence became aware of this pattern and took action to break the cycle of abuse. In therapy, she was able to grieve the loss of her marriage; however, she became profoundly depressed when she recognized how the years of violence had affected her adolescent daughter. Monique had discovered that her daughter was in an abusive peer relationship. Throughout her life, Monique had been unable to set boundaries with others, citing that she felt powerless. In her own estimation, she was attracted to her ex-husband because of his confidence and assertive nature. She believed that she lacked these traits in her own personality and took comfort in the way he directed her in her life. Monique revealed that she ran away from home at 16 and that her mother was an emotionally and physically abusive alcoholic. The years of coercive control had created a climate of terror. Monique had always felt that she had failed in her role as a daughter, and her mother vocalized her disapproval often, repeatedly calling her "stupid," "lazy," and "a waste of space." Monique married at 18 and described her husband as a controlling man who "drank too much." In her marriage, her husband's physical and emotional abuse felt all too familiar. She found it eerie how he mirrored her mother's earlier words despite having never met her. As Monique became aware of this pattern, she reflected on the

[1] A pseudonym has been used to preserve confidentiality.

pattern and surmised that it can be hard to accept love when we don't feel worthy of it. Monique believed that she was only deserving of the kind of love that felt painful, conditional, and oppressive as she had been conditioned and primed by her abusive mother to be submissive, silent, and shameful, never deeming possible her own self-sufficiency. For years, she sought approval from her mother and subsequently her husband, pining for the affection that she could never receive. As she recognized this pattern, she decided that she would never let herself fall prey to control, coercion, and arrogance again. Over time she began to feel worthy of setting boundaries and gradually educated her daughter about what respectful, safe companionship looks like.

This type of restitution in no way exonerates the perpetrator of his crimes; rather, it reaffirms the survivor's claim to moral choice in the present. This phenomenological pattern in trauma treatment demonstrates that the experience of attachment-based relational trauma in the formative years creates a vulnerability to severe emotional dysregulation along with intense feelings of despair, anxiety, shame, and mistrust of others later on in life. Therefore, clients who meet the diagnostic criteria for C-PTSD are often actively re-experiencing aspects of their early relational trauma. If left unresolved, this attachment reenactment will likely impede or play out over the course of clinical treatment.

Neuroscience of Complex Trauma

Survivors of childhood trauma with insecure attachment patterns have been found to have a higher incidence of callosal disconnection syndrome, a condition characterized by a cluster of neurological abnormalities arising from the partial or complete severing or lesioning of the corpus callosum (CC) (Applegate & Shapiro, 2005; Rinne-Albers et al., 2016). De Bellis et al. (1999) have argued that impairments to the CC resulting from complex trauma represent a preexisting vulnerability factor, predisposing individuals previously exposed to stress to developing PTSD. Classic PTSD symptoms, such as intrusive thoughts, avoidance, hyperarousal, and dissociation, have been negatively correlated with intracranial and corpus callosum volume (De Bellis et al., 1999). Thus, changes at the neurological level can heighten one's pathologic vulnerability to psychological trauma and the development of PTSD (Gilbertson et al., 2002).

Bowlby (1989) hypothesized that a child's earliest experiences with their parents lead to the development of beliefs regarding self-worth, safety, and security and the trustworthiness of others. This concept has been classically termed the "internal working model." Similarly, the Adaptive Information Processing (AIP) model explains how early formative experiences impact functioning and cognition later in life. The AIP model posits that memories of distressing experiences are dysfunctionally stored in the brain in an unmetabolized state in the memory networks that contain perceptions, negative beliefs, affect, and body sensations that arose during the experience (Shapiro, 2007; Shapiro, 2018). When an individual is traumatized, they experience strong reactions that can overwhelm the brain. As a result, distressing memories can become frozen in time, manifesting through emotional and physical distress. The unmetabolized memories, much like a "skipping disc," will replay the most distressing part of the memory, causing intrusive thoughts, shame-based cognition, and psychological reactivity that can be activated by sensitivity cues. A child who has endured numerous experiences of rejection by the attachment figure has a memory network which can be easily triggered in adulthood; this results in the development of C-PTSD and a fragmented sense of self (van der Kolk, 2015). Therefore, survivors of complex trauma will have complicated relationships with themselves and their bodies, which may be addressed compassionately through psychoeducation focused on how trauma impacts the brain (O'Shea Brown, 2020).

When an individual has distressing memories that are unmetabolized, they may be later triggered when an individual recalls the event or when the trauma survivor is exposed to sensitivity cues. The amygdala is a neural structure within the limbic system, thought to be heavily involved in integrating and making meaning of emotional information (Shapiro, 2007). The amygdala is also highly reactive to salient stimuli, including the sensations of taste, touch, and smell. This part of the brain's structure is commonly compared to an alarm, because of its heightened reactivity to emotional or threatening stimuli. Individuals with PTSD tend to demonstrate heightened amygdala volume and overexcitation within this region (Hull, 2002). As an arousal-based structure, the amygdala is likely involved in imprinting experiences of highest arousal and emotional valence. The more intense the arousal, the stronger the imprint. For instance, the smell of gun powder may trigger veterans' "imprinted memory" of a time when their life was endangered. The body can adaptively respond to these triggers by releasing hormones such as cortisol and adrenaline, to enable an effective fight-or-flight reaction.

However, if trauma is interpersonal in nature, an individual's neurobiology becomes primed to respond to interpersonal interactions that resemble the original traumatic event with fear. The brain has the remarkable ability to link a current situation with anything that looks like, feels like, smells like, or tastes like a previous threatening event (sensitivity cues). For example, if you were constantly made to feel like you were not good enough by an abusive or distant parent, later in life, this central negative cognition may become activated by a distressing event or trauma. This can result in cognitive hyperarousal or cognitive hypoarousal (see Chap. 6). Cognitive hyperarousal is characterized by hypervigilance, emotional reactivity, intrusive thoughts, and rumination (Ogden & Minton, 2000). Someone who experiences cognitive hypoarousal in response to a trauma trigger might feel numb or withdrawn. Trauma survivors often describe this as "blacking out" and/or "a fog surrounding their past." Many complex trauma survivors will report only remembering fragments of the trauma. The olfactory senses are closely tied to nostalgia—thus even if a person does not have a vivid memory of an event, they may still have the ability to tie a scent to an affective state. For example, a client may say: *The scent of patchouli makes me feel "dirty"... a creepy uncle used to wear this scent. I remember feeling uncomfortable around him, but I don't remember much from my childhood.* Or: *The sound of crunching plastic makes me feel panicked and deeply hungry; it reminds me of my childhood home...it was always infested with cockroaches and mice. I would try to feed myself but the only food in the pantry was either moldy or full of roaches.* By being curious and compassionate about a client's sensitively cue, a clinician can begin to unlock memories through sensory experiences and affective state fragments.

The hippocampus is a brain region heavily involved in the formation and storage of memories. When memories are recalled, the body or emotional sensations that accompany the memory tend to also emerge. With the passage of time, the brain integrates memories into the neocortical system, allowing for learning to occur (Stickgold, 2002). This transference often occurs during REM sleep. When a trauma is experienced, this transfer does not necessarily occur (Shapiro & Forrest, 2016). Consequentially, the adverse memory may get "stuck" or "frozen" along with the initial childlike interpretation or belief of the sensory information. Complex trauma results in re-experiencing of the painful event, signaled by nightmares and frequent enactment of the sensory responses associated with the memory. Often when an individual is recalling a traumatic event, a part of them is not aware of the present circumstances and that they are no longer at direct risk (Applegate & Shapiro, 2005).

Early experiences can directly influence emotion regulation capabilities through changes at the neural level. Consequentially the first step of trauma healing is establishing a sense of safety in the body through the promotion of successful regulation techniques (O'Shea Brown, 2021). As discussed, the phenomenological pattern of repetition compulsion in trauma treatment demonstrates that the experience of attachment-based relational trauma in the formative years creates a vulnerability to severe emotional dysregulation accompanied by intense feelings of despair, anxiety, shame, and mistrust of others later on in life. Therefore, clients who meet the diagnostic criteria for C-PTSD often actively re-experience aspects of their early relational trauma. When frequently reactivated, the trauma survivor's neurobiology will become habituated, leading to cognitive hypoarousal, which is characterized by decreased awareness, dissociation, and flat affect (Ogden & Minton, 2000). Neurobiologically speaking, the prefrontal cortex is responsible for regulatory functioning and exerts top-down control over limbic regions like the amygdala to downregulate reactivity and return functioning to baseline. Following trauma, this regulatory process can become interrupted and behaviorally manifest as irritability, withdrawal, and/or numbing (Applegate & Shapiro, 2005). The signs and symptoms of cognitive hypoarousal and dissociation will be explored more fully in Chapters 5 and 6.

Measuring Trauma in a Clinical Setting

Posttraumatic outcomes manifest differently in individuals in terms of severity, chronicity, and impact on quality of life. Therefore, the initial approach to assessment is critically important. The clinician must make an informed judgment as to what are likely to be the relevant areas of distress or dysfunction for a given client.

This clinical determination is made during the initial interview, when a traumatic event history and presenting complaints are elicited and the client's overall clinical presentation is considered (Briere & Spinazzola, 2005). This process may be assisted by a structured review of potentially traumatic events and the administration of broad-spectrum screening methods used to measure trauma. This subsequent section shall review the assessment measures: the PTSD Checklist for the DSM-5 (Weathers et al., 2013) and the International Trauma Questionnaire (ITQ) (Cloitre et al., 2018). The PTSD Checklist for DSM-5 (PCL-5) is a 20-item self-report measure that assesses the presence and severity of PTSD symptoms (see Fig. 3.1). Items on the PCL-5 correspond with DSM-5 criteria for PTSD. The PCL-5 can be used to quantify and monitor symptoms over time, to screen individuals for PTSD, and to

In the past month, how much were you bothered by:	*Not at all*	*A little bit*	*Moderately*	*Quite a bit*	*Extremely*
1. Repeated, disturbing, and unwanted memories of the stressful experience?	0	1	2	3	4
2. Repeated, disturbing dreams of the stressful experience?	0	1	2	3	4
3. Suddenly feeling or acting as if the stressful experience were actually happening again *(as if you were actually back there reliving it)*?	0	1	2	3	4
4. Feeling very upset when something reminded you of the stressful experience?	0	1	2	3	4
5. Having strong physical reactions when something reminded you of the stressful experience *(for example, heart pounding, trouble breathing, sweating)*?	0	1	2	3	4
6. Avoiding memories, thoughts, or feelings related to the stressful experience?	0	1	2	3	4
7. Avoiding external reminders of the stressful experience *(for example, people, places, conversations, activities, objects, or situations)*?	0	1	2	3	4
8. Trouble remembering important parts of the stressful experience?	0	1	2	3	4
9. Having strong negative beliefs about yourself, other people, or the world *(for example, having thoughts such as: I am bad, there is something seriously wrong with me, no one can be trusted, the world is completely dangerous)*?	0	1	2	3	4
10. Blaming yourself or someone else for the stressful experience or what happened after it?	0	1	2	3	4
11. Having strong negative feelings such as fear, horror, anger, guilt, or shame?	0	1	2	3	4
12. Loss of interest in activities that you used to enjoy?	0	1	2	3	4
13. Feeling distant or cut off from other people?	0	1	2	3	4
14. Trouble experiencing positive feelings *(for example, being unable to feel happiness or have loving feelings for people close to you)*?	0	1	2	3	4
15. Irritable behavior, angry outbursts, or acting aggressively?	0	1	2	3	4
16. Taking too many risks or doing things that could cause you harm?	0	1	2	3	4
17. Being "superalert" or watchful or on guard?	0	1	2	3	4
18. Feeling jumpy or easily startled?	0	1	2	3	4
19. Having difficulty concentrating?	0	1	2	3	4
20. Trouble falling or staying asleep?	0	1	2	3	4

Fig. 3.1 The PTSD Checklist for DSM-5 (PCL-5). (Source: Weathers et al., 2013)

assist in making a provisional or temporary diagnosis of PTSD. This measure assesses the respondent's posttraumatic stress symptoms and is designed to be administered monthly. Responders to the PCL-5 are asked to rate how bothered they have been by each item in the past month on a 5-point Likert scale ranging from 0 to 4. Items are summed to provide a total score. This is detailed in the answer key as shown in Fig. 3.2.

A provisional PTSD diagnosis can be made by treating each item rated as 2 = "Moderately" or higher as a symptom endorsed and then following the DSM-5 diagnostic rule which requires at least one Criterion B item (questions 1–5), one Criterion C item (questions 6–7), two Criterion D items (questions 8–14), and two Criterion E items (questions 15–20). A PCL-5 cutoff point of 33 appears to be a reasonable value to use for provisional PTSD diagnosis. A critique of this measurement tool is that it is self-reported; therefore, respondents may answer questions in an aspirational rather than a truthful manner. Furthermore, this scale has not been adapted to measure complex trauma. The International Trauma Questionnaire (ITQ) is a self-report designed to measure the core features of both PTSD and C-PTSD developed by Cloitre et al. (2018). The ITQ measures the six symptom clusters that correspond with *ICD-11* criteria for C-PTSD, including (i) re-experiencing of the trauma, (ii) deliberate avoidance of traumatic reminders, (iii) hypervigilance and hyperarousal, (iv) emotional regulation difficulties, (v) a persistent negative view of the self, and (vi) interpersonal problems characterized by difficulty forming and maintaining relationships with others. This self-report measure was specifically designed to assess for symptom criteria of the *ICD 11* C-PTSD (see Fig. 3.3). Therefore, it is at the cutting edge of assessment of C-PTSD at the time of this publication. The ITQ can be used to quantify and monitor symptoms over time, to screen individuals for C-PTSD, and to assist in making a provisional or temporary diagnosis. The ITQ measure assesses the respondent's post-complex trauma stress symptoms. Responders to the ITQ are asked to rate how bothered they have been by each item on a 5-point Likert scale ranging from 0 to 4. This is demonstrated along with the answer key on Fig. 3.3.

- ***Diagnostic criteria for PTSD*** require a score of ≥2 ("moderately") for at least one of two symptoms from each of the re-experiencing, avoidance, and threat clusters and at least one functional impairment item to be endorsed (≥2).
- ***Diagnostic criteria for C-PTSD*** include satisfying PTSD criteria in addition to scoring ≥2 ("moderately") for at least one symptom from each of the affective dysregulation, negative self-concept, and disturbed relationships clusters and at least one functional impairment item to be endorsed (≥2). A diagnosis of C-PTSD requires the endorsement of one of two symptoms from each of the three PTSD symptom clusters (re-experiencing in the here and now, avoidance, and sense of current threat) and one of two symptoms from each of the three Disturbances in Self-Organization (DSO) clusters: (1) affective dysregulation, (2) negative self-concept, and (3) disturbances in relationships.

Based on the *ICD-11* diagnostic rules, a diagnosis of PTSD or C-PTSD can be determined, but not both. Items are summed to provide a total score. Despite the

CRITERION	QUESTION NUMBER							TOTALS
INTRUSION SYMPTOMS B	B1 (1)	B2 (2)	B3 (3)	B4 (4)	B5 (5)			
AVOIDANCE SYMPTOMS C	C1 (6)	C2 (7)						
COGNITION & MOOD CHANGE D	D1 (8)	D2 (9)	D3 (10)	D4 (11)	D5 (12)	D6 (13)	D7 (14)	
AROUSAL & REACTIVITY E	E1 (15)	E2 (16)	E3 (17)	E4 (18)	E5 (19)	E6 (20)		
							TOTAL SCORE	

Criterion B - at least one ≥ 2 YES/NO
Criterion C - at least one ≥ 2 YES/NO
Criterion D - at least one ≥ 2 YES/NO
Criterion E - at least one ≥ 2 YES/NO

DSM5 CATEGORIES	
Mild	0-20
Moderate	20-40
Severe	40-60
Extreme	60-80

Fig. 3.2 The answer key for the PTSD Checklist for DSM-5 (PCL-5). (Source: Weathers et al., 2013)

International Trauma Questionnaire

Instructions:Please identify the experience that troubles you most and answer the questions in relation to this experience.

Brief description of the experience ______________________

When did the experience occur? (circle one)
a. less than 6 months ago
b. 6 to12 months ago
c. 1 to 5 years ago
d. 5 to 10 years ago
e. 10 to 20 years ago
f. more than 20 years ago

Below are a number of problems that people sometimes report in response to traumatic or stressful life events. Please read each item carefully, then circle one of the numbers to the right to indicate how much you have been bothered by that problem in the past month

	Not at all	*A little bit*	*Moderately*	*Quite a bit*	*Extremely*
P1. Having upsetting dreams that replay part of the experience or are clearly related to the experience?	0	1	2	3	4
P2. Having powerful images or memories that sometimes come into your mind in which you feel the experience is happening again in the here and now?	0	1	2	3	4
P3. Avoiding internal reminders of the experience (for example, thoughts, feelings, or physical sensations)?	0	1	2	3	4
P4. Avoiding external reminders of the experience (for example, people, places, conversations, objects activities, or situations)?	0	1	2	3	4
P5. Being "super-alert", watchful, or on guard?	0	1	2	3	4
P6. Feeling jumpy or easily startled?	0	1	2	3	4

In the past month have the above problems:

P7. Affected your relationships or social life?	0	1	2	3	4
P8. Affected your work or ability to work?	0	1	2	3	4
P9. Affected any other important part of your life such as parenting, or school or college work, or other important activities?	0	1	2	3	4

Fig. 3.3 The International Trauma Questionnaire. (Reprinted from Acta Psychiatrica Scandinavica, 138(6), Cloitre, M., Shevlin M., Brewin, C.R., Bisson, J.I., Roberts, N.P., Maercker, A., Karatzias, T., Hyland, P., The International Trauma Questionnaire: development of a self-report measure of ICD-11 PTSD and complex PTSD, 2018, with permission from © 2018 John Wiley & Sons A/S. Published by John Wiley & Sons Ltd.)

Below are problems that people who have had stressful or traumatic events sometimes experience. The questions refer to ways you typically feel, ways you typically think about yourself and ways you typically relate to others. Answer the following thinking about how true each statement is of you.

How true is this of you?	*Not at all*	*A little bit*	*Moderately*	*Quit a bit*	*Extremely*
C1. When I am upset, it takes me a long time to calm down	0	1	2	3	4
C2. I feel numb or emotionally shut down.	0	1	2	3	4
C3. I feel like a failure.	0	1	2	3	4
C4. I feel worthless.	0	1	2	3	4
C5. I feel distant or cut off from people.	0	1	2	3	4
C6. I find it hard to stay emotionally close to people.	0	1	2	3	4
In the past month, have the above problem in emotions, in beliefs about yourself and in relationships;					
C7. Created concern or distress about your relationships or social life?	0	1	2	3	4
C8. Affected your work or ability to work?	0	1	2	3	4
C9. Affected any other important parts of your life such as parenting, or school or college work, or other important activities?	0	1	2	3	4

Fig. 3.3 (continued)

ITQ having been recently developed, early research has supported its psychometric properties in multiple trauma-exposed samples (Cloitre et al., 2018; Hyland et al., 2018; Karatzias et al., 2016). However, a critique of this measure is that it is self-reported; therefore, questions may be answered in an aspirational manner. At this time, it is not endorsed by the DSM; however, it is hoped that this will change.

Both the PCL-5 and the ITQ are helpful resources in measuring trauma symptoms. However, when administered alongside the Adverse Childhood Experiences Questionnaire (explored in Chap. 4) and in conjunction with the Scale of Dissociative Experiences (explored in Chap. 5), this can provide a more accurate picture of symptoms derived from a past history of chronic, prolonged relational trauma in addition to identifying triggering stimuli.

Summary

Childhood trauma, including abuse and neglect, is a major public health concern. It poses a challenge that has the potential to be largely resolved by appropriate prevention and intervention. An insidious part of complex trauma is that it usually begins in the home and a vast majority of those responsible for child maltreatment are the children's own parent(s). By sensitively attuning to your clients' needs and understanding the origins and impacts of their complex trauma, effective treatment planning can commence. The subsequent chapter shall explore the role of dysfunctional family systems in the development of C-PTSD.

Questions and Activities for Discussion and Further Reflection

1. What are the core differences between C-PTSD and PTSD?
2. List and describe the challenges of working with a client with C-PTSD.
3. What are the implications of complex trauma on one's parenting, relationships, and the clinical relationship?

Thought Experiment

Research exploring the differences in individual- and cluster-level posttraumatic stress symptoms indicate that trauma may manifest differently cross-culturally. Marshall, Schell, and Miles (2009) found that in a sample group comprised of Hispanic, non-Hispanic Caucasian, and African American survivors of sudden physical injury, there was a variation in the manifestation of PTSD symptoms cross-culturally. The study found that the Hispanic group reported higher levels of overall posttraumatic distress along with different patterns of symptoms, i.e., hypervigilance versus sleep disturbance and numbing. Subsequent studies researching the cross-cultural manifestation of posttraumatic stress symptoms have been inconsistent.

After reading this article, host a class discussion to explore the following question: Is the manifestation of posttraumatic stress symptoms different and unique to each culture? This conversation can be guided through the following themes: cultural norms, expression versus suppression, transgenerational trauma, language, and mental health stigma.

Exercise

1. Class Discussion Prompt: Reflect on the difference between single incident trauma and layered complex trauma. How would this shape behavioral patterns, for instance, in addiction, sexuality, risk behaviors, and disordered eating patterns?
2. Self-administer *the International Trauma Questionnaire* (ITQ) – Any personal reflections on the questionnaire are welcome in a smaller group discussion (3–5 students per group).

References

American Psychiatric Association. (1980). *Diagnostic and statistical manual of mental disorders* (3rd ed.). Washington, DC: American Psychiatric Publishing.

American Psychiatric Association. (2013). *Diagnostic and statistical manual of mental disorders* (5th ed.). Washington, DC: American Psychiatric Publishing.

Applegate, J. S., & Shapiro, J. R. (2005). *Neurobiology for clinical social work: Theory and practice*. New York, NY: W.W. Norton & Co.

Bowlby, J. (1989). The role of attachment in personality development and psychopathology. In S. I. Greenspan & G. H. Pollack (Eds.), *The course of life: Vol. 1. Infancy* (pp. 119–136). Madison, CT: International Universities Press.

Briere, J., & Spinazzola, J. (2005). Phenomenology and psychological assessment of complex posttraumatic states. *Journal of Traumatic Stress, 18*(5), 401–412.

Centers for Disease Control and Prevention, National Center for Injury Prevention and Control, Division of Violence Prevention. (2014, May). *The Adverse Childhood Experiences (ACE) Study. cdc.gov*. Atlanta, Georgia. Archived from the original on 27 December 2015.

Cloitre, M., Courtois, C. A., Charuvastra, A., Carapezza, R., Stolbach, B. C., & Green, B. L. (2011). Treatment of complex PTSD: Results of the ISTSS expert clinician survey on best practices. *Journal of Traumatic Stress, 24*, 615–627.

Cloitre, M., Shevlin, M., Brewin, C. R., Bisson, J. I., Roberts, N. P., Maercker, A., … Hyland, P. (2018). The international trauma questionnaire: Development of a self-report measure of ICD-11 PTSD and complex PTSD. *Acta Psychiatrica Scandinavica, 138*, 536–546. https://doi.org/10.1111/acps.12956

Collins, N. L., & Read, S. J. (1990). Adult attachment, working models, and relationship quality in dating couples. *Journal of Personality and Social Psychology, 58*, 644–663.

Courtois, C. A. (1988). *Healing the incest wound: Adult survivors in therapy*. W W Norton & Co.

De Bellis, M. D., Keshavan, M., Clark, D. B., Casey, B. J., Giedd, J., Boring, A. M., … Bennett, A. E. (1999). Research award. Developmental traumatology, part II: Brain development. *Biological Psychiatry, 45*, 1271–1284.

Fairbairn, W. R. D. (1943). The repression and the return of bad objects (with special reference to the 'war neuroses'). *British Journal of Medical Psychology, 19*, 327–341. https://doi.org/10.1111/j.2044-8341.1943.tb00328.x

Felitti, V. J., Anda, R. F., Nordenberg, D., Williamson, D. F., Spitz, A. M., Edwards, V., … Marks, J. S. (1998). Relationship of childhood abuse and household dysfunction to many of the leading causes of death in adultsThe adverse childhood experiences (ACE) study. *American Journal of Preventive Medicine, 14*, 245–258.

Freud, S. (1914). *Remembering, repeating and working-through (Further recommendations on the technique of psycho-analysis II)*. The standard edition of the complete psychological works of Sigmund Freud, volume XII (1911–1913): The Case of Schreber, Papers on Technique and Other Works, pp. 145–156.

Gilbertson, M. W., Shenton, M. E., Ciszewski, A., Kasai, K., Lasko, N. B., Orr, S. P., & Pitman, R. K. (2002). Smaller hippocampal volume predicts pathologic vulnerability to psychological trauma. *Nature Neuroscience, 5*(11), 1242–1247. https://doi.org/10.1038/nn958

Giourou, E., Skokou, M., Andrew, S. P., Alexopoulou, K., Gourzis, P., & Jelastopulu, E. (2018). Complex posttraumatic stress disorder: The need to consolidate a distinct clinical syndrome or to reevaluate features of psychiatric disorders following interpersonal trauma. *World Journal of Psychiatry, 8*(1), 12–19. https://doi.org/10.5498/wjp.v8.i1.12

Granqvist, P., Sroufe, L. A., Dozier, M., Hesse, E., Steele, M., van IJzendoorn, M., & Duschinsky, R. (2017). Disorganized attachment in infancy: A review of the phenomenon and its implications for clinicians and policy-makers. *Attachment & Human Development, 19*(6), 534–558. https://doi.org/10.1080/14616734.2017.1354040

Grant, L. (2020). Post-Vietnam syndrome: Psychiatry, anti-war politics, and the reconstitution of the Vietnam veteran. *Rhetoric of Health & Medicine, 3*(2), 189–219.

Herman, J. L. (1992). *Trauma and recovery: The aftermath of violence*. New York, NY: Basic Books.
Hull, A. M. (2002). Neuroimaging findings in post-traumatic stress disorder. Systematic review. *The British Journal of Psychiatry: The Journal of Mental Science, 181*, 102–110.
Hyland, P., Ceannt, R., Daccache, F., Abou Daher, R., Sleiman, J., Gilmore, B., Byrne, S., Shevlin, M., Murphy, J., & Vallières, F. (2018). Are posttraumatic stress disorder (PTSD) and complex-PTSD distinguishable within a treatment-seeking sample of Syrian refugees living in Lebanon?. Global mental health (Cambridge, England), 5, e14. https://doi.org/10.1017/gmh.2018.2
Jones, E. (2010). Shell Shock at Maghull and the Maudsley: The origins of psychological medicine. *Journal of the History of Medicine and Allied Sciences, 65*, 368–395.
Karatzias, T., Shevlin, M., Fyvie, C., Hyland, P., Efthymiadou, E., Wilson, D., & Cloitre, M. (2016). ICD-11 Posttraumatic Stress Disorder (PTSD) and Complex Posttraumatic Stress Disorder (CPTSD): factorial structure of a new self-report scale (ICD-TQ). *Journal of Anxiety Disorders, 44*, 73–79.
Marshall, G. N., Schell, T. L., & Miles, J. N. V. (2009). Ethnic differences in posttraumatic distress: Hispanics' symptoms differ in kind and degree. *Journal of Consulting and Clinical Psychology, 77*, 1169–1178. https://doi.org/10.1037/a0017721
McNally, R. J. (2006). Cognitive abnormalities in post-traumatic stress disorder. *Trends in Cognitive Sciences (Regul. Ed.), 10*, 271–277. https://doi.org/10.1016/j.tics.2006.04.007
Myers, C. S. (1916). Contributions to the study of shell shock, being an account of certain cases treated by hypnosis. *Lancet, 1*, 65–66.
O'Shea Brown, G. (2020). Internal family systems informed eye movement desensitization and reprocessing: An integrative technique for treatment of complex posttraumatic stress disorder. *International Body Psychotherapy Journal, 19*(2).
O'Shea Brown, G. (2021). Reflections on providing virtual eye movement desensitization and reprocessing therapy in the wake of COVID-19: Survival through adaptation. In C. Tosone (Ed.), *Shared trauma, shared resilience during a pandemic: Social work in the time of COVID-19*. Cham, Switzerland: Springer.
Ogden, P., & Minton, K. (2000). Sensorimotor psychotherapy: One method for processing traumatic memory. *Traumatology, 6*(3), 149–173. https://doi.org/10.1177/153476560000600302
Rinne-Albers, M. A., van der Werff, S. J., van Hoof, M. J., van Lang, N. D., Lamers-Winkelman, F., Rombouts, S. A., … van der Wee, N. J. (2016). Abnormalities of white matter integrity in the corpus callosum of adolescents with PTSD after childhood sexual abuse: A DTI study. *European Child & Adolescent Psychiatry, 25*(8), 869–878. https://doi.org/10.1007/s00787-015-0805-2
Rutter, M. (2007). Resilience, competence and coping. *Child Abuse & Neglect, 31*(3), 205–209.
Shakespeare, W. (1564–1616). Henry IV, part 1. [London]: London.
Shapiro, F. (2007). EMDR, adaptive information processing, and case conceptualization. *Journal of EMDR Practice and Research, 1*(2), 68–87. https://doi.org/10.1891/1933-3196.1.2.68
Shapiro, F. (2014). The role of eye movement desensitization and reprocessing (EMDR) therapy in medicine: Addressing the psychological and physical symptoms stemming from adverse life experience. *The Permanente Journal, 18*, 71–77. https://doi.org/10.7812/TPP/13-098
Shapiro, F. (2018). *Eye movement desensitization and reprocessing (EMDR) therapy: Basic principles, protocols, and procedures* (3rd ed.). New York, NY: Guilford Press.
Shapiro, F., & Forrest, M. S. (2016). *EMDR: Breakthrough therapy for overcoming anxiety, stress & trauma*. New York, NY: Basic Books.
Slavich, G. M., & Auerbach, R. P. (2018). Stress and its sequelae: Depression, suicide, inflammation, and physical illness. In J. N. Butcher & J. M. Hooley (Eds.), *APA handbook of psychopathology, Vol. 1: Psychopathology: Understanding, assessing, and treating adult mental disorders* (pp. 375–402). Washington, DC: American Psychological Association.
Stickgold, R. (2002). EMDR: A putative neurobiological mechanism of action. *The Journal of Clinical Psychiatry, 58*(1), 61–75.

Takin, S., & Hendrix, H. (2011). *Wired for love: How understanding your partner's brain and attachment style can help you defuse conflict and build a secure relationship*. Oakland, CA: New Harbringer Publications.

van der Kolk, B., Roth, S., Pelcovitz, D., Sunday, S., & Spinazzola, J. J. (2005). Disorders of extreme stress: The empirical foundation of a complex adaptation to trauma. *Journal of Trauma Stress, 18*(5), 389–399.

van der Kolk, B. A. (2005). Developmental trauma disorder: Toward a rational diagnosis for children with complex trauma histories. *Psychiatric Annals, 35*(5), 401–408.

van der Kolk, B. A. (2015). *The body keeps the score: Brain, mind and body in the healing of trauma*. New York, NY: Viking Press.

van der Kolk, B. A., McFarlane, A., & Weisaeth, L. (1996). *Traumatic stress*. New York, NY: Guilford Press.

Weathers, F. W., Litz, B. T., Keane, T. M., Palmieri, P. A., Marx, B. P., & Schnurr, P. P. (2013). *The PTSD checklist for* DSM-5 *(PCL-5)*. Scale available from the National Center for PTSD at www.ptsd.va.gov

World Health Organization [WHO] (2018). The ICD-11 for mortality and morbidity statistics. Retrieved from https://icd-who-int.proxy.library.nyu.edu/browse11/lm/en

Chapter 4
Dysfunctional Family Systems

Many people hope that once they leave the dysfunction of their family home, they will leave their childhood problems behind. However, adult children of dysfunctional families have been found to develop deficits in problem-solving communication in addition to establishing and maintaining trust in close relationships (Harrington & Metzler, 1997; Hinz, 1990; McKenna & Pickens, 1983; Webb, Post, Robinson, & Moreland, 1992). The experience of trauma or maltreatment in the formative years creates a vulnerability to severe emotional dysregulation along with intense feelings of despair, anxiety, shame, and mistrust of others later on in life. In past studies, adult children of dysfunctional families have been categorized on the basis of the presence of a traumatic event(s) such as abuse, addiction, divorce, or death of a parent (Baker & Williamson, 1989; Fisher, Jenkins, Harrison, & Jesch, 1993; Jenkins, Fisher, & Harrison, 1993). In order to understand how developmental trauma informs identity and behavioral patterns, it is important to review the theoretical underpinning of dysfunctional family systems.

This chapter will first provide a description of what constitutes a dysfunctional family system, before exploring how dysfunction can lead to pathological accommodation. The role of communication deviance and behavioral abnormalities within the family system shall be reviewed. Following this review, this chapter will evaluate current research exploring the impact that adverse childhood experiences (ACEs) have on identity, adult relationships, and social functioning. Finally, the chapter will explore how dysfunction within a family system can be measured using the ACE Questionnaire as a clinical tool.

G. O'Shea Brown, *Healing Complex Posttraumatic Stress Disorder*, Essential Clinical Social Work Series, https://doi.org/10.1007/978-3-030-61416-4_4

Dysfunctional Family Systems and Pathological Accommodation

A dysfunctional family is one in which conflict, misbehavior, and instability are present. Within a dysfunctional family system where abuse and/or neglect is present, other family members are often forced to accommodate and enable destructive behaviors. *Household dysfunction* applies to any home in which substance abuse, divorce, mental illness, suicidal activity, caretaker violence, or criminality/incarceration is present (Centers for Disease Control and Prevention, 2014). Pathological accommodation refers to ways of being that function unconsciously to preserve a needed attachment when that bond has been traumatically threatened (Brandchaft, 2007). Most often pathological accommodation occurs when the relational needs of a child are unmet through pervasive misattunement and/or hostile reactions from the primary caregiver (Doctors, 2017; Brandchaft, 2007).

Black (1981) identified three "family laws" which govern substance-dependent family systems: (a) do not talk, (b) do not trust, and (c) do not feel. Though this model was designed to understand family systems where addiction is a presenting issue, it can be applied to all dysfunctional family systems. In order to adapt to survive, children reared in such dysfunctional environments learn coping mechanisms or roles to protect themselves from fear and hurt (Wegscheider, 1981). Black (1981) suggested that it is difficult to learn how to trust when promises are frequently broken and reality is often distorted, a pattern known as "reality shifting." Examples of dysfunctional family systems include:

- One or both parents exert a strong authoritarian control over the children. Often these families rigidly adhere to particular beliefs in the religious, political, financial, and/or personal realms. Compliance with role expectations and with rules is expected without any flexibility.
- One or both parents have compulsive behavior(s), for example, an addiction to substances, sex, gambling, or overwork, which have strong influences on the other family members.
- One or both parents use the threat or application of physical violence as a means of control.
- Domestic violence is present within the home between the parents, or toward siblings, including emotional abuse and physical abuse.
- One or both parents exploit the children and treat them as possessions whose primary purpose is to respond to the physical and/or emotional needs of adults (e.g., the parentified child is caring for the parents and/or their siblings due to parental illness or mental health complications).
- One or both parents are unable to provide, or threaten to withdraw, financial or basic physical care for their children.

Wegscheider (1981) developed the family role identification theory that has become the primary model for researchers and clinicians addressing the impacts of dysfunctional family systems. Though this model was primarily developed to help clinicians understand the internal dynamics of families where substance dependency was an issue, it can be applied to a wide context of stress-filled familial contexts. Jenkins et al. (1993) noted that there may be other dynamics besides addiction that contribute to rigid role behaviors, such as physical abuse, sexual abuse, divorce, or the death of a parent. Wegscheider identified four core roles or behavioral patterns of children from such dysfunctional family systems: *(a) the hero, (b) the lost child, (c) the mascot*, and *(d) the scapegoat* (as shown in Fig. 4.1).

According to Wegscheider (1981), the *hero child* is a role played by individuals who attempt to appease other family members and act in ways that look good; they often seek approval through their achievements and responsible behavior, perhaps surmising that academia and accomplishment are more stable, predictable, and reliable sources of external validation than what is available to them at home. However, the hero tends to base much of their sense of self on their abilities to achieve. As a result, they can develop internalized guilt, shame-based cognition, and an intense fear of failing, in addition to lacking personal boundaries with other family members, especially their parents (Wegscheider, 1981). As the parents in a dysfunctional family home are too preoccupied with their own needs to be there for the children, the hero will often step in for them, assuming the role of the "parentified child." The hero child can become a source of pride to the family ("We are not so bad because this child turned out so well – we must be doing something right"). The hero child is prone to perfectionism, which causes tension and hypervigilance in their own

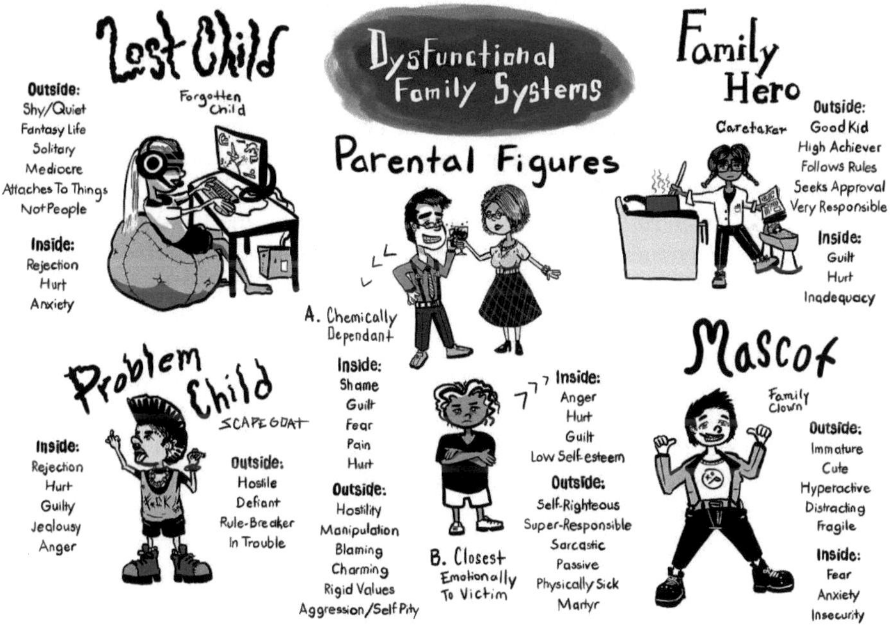

Fig. 4.1 "The family role identification theory" (Wegscheider, 1981). (Credit: Illustration commissioned from A.R. Illustration: Arillustration.art)

lives, hampering their capacity to tolerate pleasure activities, demonstrate creativity, or engage in play. They tend to be most comfortable when at work, in control, or achieving something, a tendency which can become overwhelming and unhealthy.

The *lost child*, often referred to as the "unseen child" or the "passive child," can go unnoticed in the system; as a result, this child harbors a deep sense of loneliness. The lost child has a tendency to avoid personal interaction and represses emotions. They can appear to be shy, quiet, and withdrawn toward family members and others. As a result, they are often ignored and feel deeply unheard and isolated. Consequently, the lost child often develops the behavioral pattern of a loner; instead of connecting with others, they learn to repress their emotions and seek comfort in animals, material possessions, or even crafts. The lost child has surmised that interpersonal relationships are scary and unpredictable; however, focusing attention on non-humans or objects feels like a safe way to foster a sense of connection and relationship. Parents of the lost child may reassure themselves, "At least we don't have worry about this child." However, as a result of the parent's pervasive lack of attunement and interest in their children's needs, it becomes very difficult for the "lost child" to connect with others, self-advocate, and share opinions.

The *mascot child* typically expresses the repressed emotions of other members of the family, assuming the role of the clown or jester in the family system. Aware of the building tensions within the dysfunctional family household, the mascot child attempts to find a way to dispel nervous energy in a positive way. The mascot child, similar to the lost child, seeks to emotionally disengage from the family system, albeit in very different ways. The mascot utilizes comic relief to navigate away from family issues and to conceal their true feelings of inadequacy, emotional distress, and underlying fear. As a result of their continuous denial of personal needs and emotions, the mascot child can develop into a passively compliant adult, reliant on others to lead them and make choices on their behalf. This mascot role can lead to immature behaviors, attention seeking, and difficulties in establishing autonomy and self-confidence.

Finally, the *scapegoat child* is a role often played by the child who opposes familial values and opinions and acts directly against the accepted norms of the family in a defiant way. They are often referred to as the "black sheep" because of their impulsivity and aggression. The scapegoat opposes parents' emotional expectations and often engages in risky behaviors. In many ways, the scapegoat serves as a "release valve": they become the central bearer of stress within the dysfunctional family system and are forced to assume the blame for all that is wrong with the wider family system. Parents within the dysfunctional family system will often avoid a sense of accountability for their own maladaptive behaviors or thoughts by focusing on the perceived flaws of the scapegoat child. On the inside the scapegoat child harbors feelings of shame and inadequacy due to the pervasive rejection and criticism they absorb from the family system and beyond. The scapegoat child can develop into an adult who engages in risk behaviors, promiscuity, and addiction which can lead to suffering.

Wegscheider (1981) explains that these roles are developed and adhered to by individuals as coping strategies in an adverse environment. Often children will hold more than one role at a time or may vacillate between aspects of two roles in an attempt to navigate their sense of self. Sometimes the hero and the scapegoat switch roles over time. In addition, there may be more than one of each role within a family system. Buelow (1994) has proposed that as familial interactions become more dysfunctional, the roles of hero, lost child, mascot, and scapegoat can become more rigid; conversely, the healthier the family system, the less rigid the roles. The thoughts, feelings, or behaviors associated with a role can shape the personality, which can become less flexible and adaptable over time. Herman (1992) cautions that the personality formed in the environment of coercive control or neglect is not well adapted to adult life. These rigid role behaviors at first facilitate coping, but later in life they can create personal and interpersonal difficulties (Black, 1981; Herman, 1992; Wegscheider, 1981). Adult children of dysfunctional family homes are left with fundamental problems in basic trust, autonomy, and initiative.

There is a great deal of variability in how often dysfunctional interactions and behaviors occur in families and in the kinds and the severity of dysfunction. However, when patterns like the above are the norm rather than the exception, they systematically foster abuse and/or neglect of children. The role of pathological accommodation is a trauma response to protect against the wounds of relational trauma; however, when one is pervasively operating in survival mode, they can become alienated from their true authentic self. Subsequently in this chapter, we will discuss communication deviance and abnormal behavioral patterns which often present within the dysfunctional family system.

Communication Deviance and Behavioral Abnormalities

Abnormalities in communication and behaviors are highly characteristic of the emotional abuse that occurs within dysfunctional family systems. Communication deviance is a term used to describe confusing language which is ambiguous, contradictory, and difficult to understand (Ditton, Green, & Singer, 1987). Features of communication deviance include commitment problems, referent problems, language anomalies, disruptions, and contradictory sequences (Ditton et al., 1987). Conversely, clear communication involves the establishment of joint attention, topic focus, clear referent, and shared meaning between parent and child during a communication exchange (Rosengren, Behrend, & Perlmutter, 1993). At a deeper level, shared meaning is indicative that family members are facilitated in understanding the different values, beliefs, and emotions that each member has and associates with particular words. Researchers have hypothesized that, over time, parental communication clarity may influence the development of children's learning, ability to trust, and problem-solving communication (Rosengren et al., 1993; Singer, Wynne, & Toohey, 1978). Clear communication creates the foundation for relational trust; however, many dysfunctional families are unable to listen to one another, and consequently individual members often feel misunderstood, unimportant, and unheard in the context of the family system. (Black, 1981; Wegscheider, 1981). Without clear communication, passive-aggressive behaviors, tension, and mistrust develop, all of which erode familial bonds and violate the trust and boundaries of family members. This chapter subsection reviews terms that discuss and provide an understanding of communication deviance and abnormal behavioral patterns which are often present within the dysfunctional family system.

Terms describing communication deviance and abnormal behavioral patterns	
Covert incest/the parentified child	Covert incest, also known as emotional incest, is a type of abuse in which a parent looks to their child for the emotional support that would be normally provided by another adult.
Double-bind messages	The double-bind message described by Bateson, Jackson, Haley, and Weakland (1963) is a message containing two conflicting statements, each of which negates the other. An example of a double-bind message is being forced to falsely confess to an accusation and be punished or deny the accusation, be accused of lying, and be punished anyway. Children who are physically abused are told to be silent but also told to ask for help by their abusers, who will likely punish them for any perceived shortcomings. The dilemma posed is that all actions lead to a negative outcome for the recipient. The double-bind message always places the recipient in the wrong: They are asked to be serious and not serious, work more and work less, be more attractive and less attractive, ask for help but not be needy. Double-bind messages are often utilized as a form of control via covert coercion by dysfunctional parents toward a child. This can occur when parents intermittently ask a child to enable their compulsive behaviors and support their recovery. Another example would be a parent asking a child to be open and honest, but then denying them their truth (with regard to sexual orientation, gender expression, emotional needs, etc.). The child is in trouble both for being truthful and for keeping secrets. This is highly emotionally abusive, as the confusing nature of the statement constitutes a "no win" manipulation whereby the recipient is encouraged to be passive and compliant in the relationship.
Walking on eggshells	The term "walking on eggshells" is often used by individuals who describe a childhood of tiptoeing around a parent's unpredictable behaviors and polarizing mood swings. They may describe intermittently experiencing rejection and/or preferential treatment. The instability of the parent may be due to mental health issues, addiction, or other underlying vulnerabilities.

Terms describing communication deviance and abnormal behavioral patterns	
Projective identification	Klein (1946) coined the term "projective identification" to describe a primitive defense mechanism in which an individual projects unwanted thoughts or feelings onto another and identifies the projected material as belonging to another. We are familiar with the concept of the schoolyard bully who, struggling to cope with their feelings of inadequacy, projects their internalized shame onto others via name-calling and criticisms. This same dynamic can occur between dysfunctional, unwell parents toward their unsuspecting children. For example, a child has a sleepover at a friend's house, and the parent feels lonely and inadequate in their absence. Rather than process their separation anxiety, they project their feelings of inadequacy onto the child by telling the child that the child is selfish and/or inadequate. Projective identification is connected to the detailed reality shifting (described later in this section). Projective identification is a defense mechanism in which the individual projects qualities that are unacceptable to the self onto another person, and that person internalizes the projected qualities. For instance, a wife has been having an extramarital affair. She has been experiencing feelings of guilt and shame due to the secrecy. However, rather than process these unwanted emotions, she projects her feelings of insecurity onto her unsuspecting spouse whom she accuses of dishonesty and infidelity. Projective identification is an unconscious phantasy in which aspects of the self or an internal object are split off and attributed to an external object. The projected aspects may be felt by the projector to be either good or bad. This can create toxic stress within relationships and family systems.
Loyalty bind	Alliances and conflicts emerge in all family systems; however, within the dysfunctional family system, loyalty binds are especially hazardous to a child's well-being. A child may be forced to take sides in conflicts between parents or between parents and siblings. This can often result in the child being restricted from full and direct communication with other family members or having to keep secrets as a demonstration of loyalty. An example is a child discovering adultery or incest and being warned by the parent that if they reveal the secret it will be their fault that the family is torn apart. The result is that the child lives with a deep sense of distrust of others and shame-based cognition.
Triangulation	Triangulation as described by Bowen (1976) is a two-person emotional system that is unstable and that, when under stress, forms itself into a three-person system or triangle. In this relational triangle communication pattern, one person will not communicate directly with another person, instead using a third person to relay communication to the second. Triangulation is a manipulation tactic and also refers to covert controlling communication to engineer rivalry between two people or "playing one against another" (Aponte & Van Deusen, 1981). For example, a child and father in chronic conflict might both persistently compete for the support of the mother, who in turn tries to balance her favor between them. The emotional intensity of such coalitions often contributes to physical and emotional symptomatology in the child. This is due to the level of stress experienced in an environment devoid of trust, transparency, and harmony.
Coercion	Coercion within a dysfunctional family system usually involves one or both of the parents enforcing an excessive structure and placing demands on their children's time, choice of friends, or behavior.

Terms describing communication deviance and abnormal behavioral patterns	
Enmeshment	Enmeshment is a term used to describe families with extremely diffuse boundaries, where self-sufficiency is compromised (Williams & Hiebert, 2001). Adult children from enmeshed families typically struggle with an exaggerated or inappropriate level of guilt and shame-based cognition. Within an enmeshed family, the parent becomes dependent upon a child to fulfill their emotional needs. In the context of such families, parents may be inappropriately intrusive, overly involved, and protective. Though there is a sense of connection and collective support within an enmeshed family system, there is often pressure to obey high demands for loyalty or conformity to the family, and consequently development of individual autonomy and the ability to set boundaries are both greatly inhibited.
Pathological accommodation	Within a dysfunctional family system where abuse and/or neglect is present, other family members are often forced to accommodate and enable destructive behaviors. Pathological accommodation refers to ways of being that function unconsciously to preserve a needed attachment when that bond has been traumatically threatened (Brandchaft, 2007). Most often pathological accommodation occurs when the relational needs of a child are unmet through pervasive misattunement and hostile reactions from the primary caregiver (Doctors, 2017; Brandchaft, 2007).
Reality shifting	Black (1981) suggested that it is difficult to learn how to trust when promises are frequently broken and reality is often distorted, in a pattern known as "reality shifting." Reality shifting is colloquially known as "gaslighting," a term derived from the 1938 British play *Gaslight*, which conveys the story of a husband who causes his wife to doubt her own perceptions of reality with manipulative techniques. Gaslighting is a form of manipulation where the perpetrator attempts to convince someone that their thoughts, perceptions, or beliefs are mistaken; often it is seen as part of a wider constellation of abuse (Riggs & Bartholomaeus, 2018). Within the dysfunctional family system, the experience of reality shifting can be an unconscious and covert process, in which what is said contradicts what is actually happening. An example of reality shifting would be a parent denying that a child was abused despite having actually observed the abuse. Another example would be the experience of a transgender teen attempting to find their identity in the context of a family system that denies that identity's existence (Riggs & Bartholomaeus, 2018).

To understand the imprint of complex trauma, the foundational step is to earn the trust of the survivor. The above terms are intended to validate and affirm the experiences of adult survivors of complex trauma and provide them with an enhanced understanding of their experience (O'Shea Brown, 2021). From there we can begin to provide them with the knowledge, psychoeducation, and terminology to understand what they have survived, and in doing so, we strive to create for them a place of safety. Many survivors of childhood abuse have memories of their past disclosures of abuse being ignored and discounted and perhaps even blamed on them by family members (O'Shea Brown, 2020b). As their empathic witness, the clinician must, during the history taking segment of the treatment plan, learn family names and behavioral patterns and help the client to identify the roles they were forced to assume during those formative years of childhood adversity.

Adverse Childhood Experiences

The Centers for Disease Control and Prevention (CDC) defines adverse childhood experiences as those experiences, such as abuse and household dysfunction, that occur before the age of 18 and cause extreme distress resulting in long-term medical, mental health, and behavioral implications (Centers for Disease Control and Prevention, 2014). The Adverse Childhood Experiences Study (ACES) sought to understand how adversity in the formative years goes on to impede healthy development and wellness in adulthood (Felitti et al., 1998). Trauma, as defined by a person's subjective assignment of meaning, can result from a variety of experiences, and the impact of these experiences can be conceptualized as stemming from a single event or multiple events resultant from clusters of repeated traumas termed adverse childhood experiences (i.e., complex trauma as discussed in Chap. 3).

This study found that adult survivors of clustered adverse childhood experiences went on to develop high-risk maladaptive behaviors, difficulty in establishing and maintaining healthy relationships, and mental distress, in addition to poor physical health (Felitti et al., 1998). By administering the ACE Questionnaire (ACE-Q) (Box 4.1), a clinician can begin to understand and gather information regarding potentially traumatic events that occurred in childhood (e.g., experiencing violence, abuse, or neglect; witnessing violence in the home or community; and/or having a family member attempt or die by suicide). The ACE-Q also includes questions exploring aspects of a child's environment that can undermine their sense of safety, stability, and bonding, such as growing up in a household with substance misuse, mental health problems, or instability due to parental separation or incarceration of a household member. The ACES found that the higher someone's ACE score – the more types of childhood adversity a person experienced. ACEs are linked to chronic health problems, mental illness, and substance misuse in adulthood. The study found that most people (64%) have at least one ACE; 12% of the population has an ACE score of 4 or higher. Having an ACE score of 4 nearly doubles the risk of heart disease and cancer. Poignantly, this study also identified that there was a high prevalence for suicidality and an impulse to ritualistically, compulsively comfort-seek, leading to addiction among individuals with a high ACE score (CDC, 2014; Felitti et al., 1998). Having an ACE score of 4 or higher increases the likelihood of becoming an alcoholic by 700% and the risk of attempted suicide by 1200% (Felitti et al., 1998; CDC, 2014). ACEs can also negatively impact education and job opportunities.

Ritualized, compulsive comfort-seeking—what traditionalists call addiction—is a relatively common response to the adversity experienced in childhood, emerging as a coping behavior for survivors who were never taught healthy alternatives for managing stress when they were young (Derefinko et al., 2019). This will be explored more fully in Chap. 6, which covers the impact of trauma on the body. Over the two decades since the development and first use of the ACE-Q in a large population study, research using the ACE-Q and its variants has repeatedly demonstrated a linkage between ACEs and increased risk of acquiring a wide range of psychiatric disorders, addictions, and medical (multi-organ) illnesses in adulthood that ultimately involve high-cost medical care and premature death (Brown et al., 2010; Zarse et al., 2019).

Survivors of adverse childhood experience also fared poorly in academic achievement and overall employment stability over the course of a lifetime. To attempt to pursue a goal that society has made unattainable is to condemn oneself to a state of perpetual dissatisfaction (O'Shea Brown, 2020a). One cannot survive repeated disappointments of experience indefinitely. A critique of the ACE-Q is that it lacks questions pertaining to childhood experiences of homelessness, racism, being transgender, and being an immigrant. These adverse experiences are overlooked in the questionnaire. Therefore, it is recommended that the tool be updated to reflect the adversity that comes with intersectionality and displacement. For example, one area of expansion may be the inclusion of a question pertaining to a child's exposure to racism, discrimination, stigma, or minority stress. The inclusion of the following question may enhance the research of the long-term impacts of the childhood experience of racism and discrimination: *have you ever been treated differently or judged unfairly because of your race or ethnicity?* Aside from personal/interpersonal racism, the experience of institutional/systemic racism can adversely impact health-seeking behaviors, sense of belonging, acceptance, and emotional well-being. Therefore, it is hoped that the ACE-Q continues to grow and evolve to measure, affirm, and protect all children from personal and systemic adversity.

Measuring Adverse Childhood Experiences in a Clinical Setting

The ACE Questionnaire is a self-administered instrument that includes ten questions to which the individual will give a Yes or No answer. When scoring, each "Yes" answer will be given one (1) point. These points will be tallied to determine the individual's ACE score. Administering the ACE-Q in a clinical setting can aid the clinician in facilitating the client to identify traumatic experiences in their past. In clinical settings, the results of the survey can be used as a starting point for effective treatment planning and to educate clients about the impact of traumatic childhood experiences on their health and well-being. This questionnaire can be viewed in its entirety in Box 4.1.

Box 4.1 Adverse Childhood Experiences Questionnaire (Centers for Disease Control and Prevention, n.d.)

Finding Your ACE Score

While you were growing up, during your first 18 years of life:

(continued)

Box 4.1 (continued)

1. Did a parent or other adult in the household *often or very often*…

   Swear at you, insult you, put you down, or humiliate you?
   or
   Act in a way that made you afraid that you might be physically hurt?

   Yes No If yes enter 1 ________

2. Did a parent or other adult in the household *often or very often*…

   Push, grab, slap, or throw something at you?
   or
   Ever hit you so hard that you had marks or were injured?

   Yes No If yes enter 1 ________

3. Did an adult or person at least 5 years older than you *ever*…

   Touch or fondle you or have you touch their body in a sexual way?
   or
   Attempt or actually have oral, anal, or vaginal intercourse with you?

   Yes No If yes enter 1 ________

4. Did you *often or very often* feel that …

   No one in your family loved you or thought you were important or special?
   or
   Your family didn't look out for each other, feel close to each other, or support each other?

   Yes No If yes enter 1 ________

5. Did you *often or very often* feel that …

   You didn't have enough to eat, had to wear dirty clothes, and had no one to protect you?
   or
   Your parents were too drunk or high to take care of you or take you to the doctor if you needed it?

   Yes No If yes enter 1 ________

6. Were your parents *ever* separated or divorced?

   Yes No If yes enter 1 ________

7. Was your mother or stepmother:

   Often or very often pushed, grabbed, slapped, or had something thrown at her?
   or
   Sometimes, often, or very often kicked, bitten, hit with a fist, or hit with something hard?
   or
   Ever repeatedly hit at least a few minutes or threatened with a gun or knife?

   Yes No If yes enter 1 ________

8. Did you live with anyone who was a problem drinker or alcoholic or who used street drugs?

   Yes No If yes enter 1 ________

9. Was a household member depressed or mentally ill, or did a household member attempt suicide?

   Yes No If yes enter 1 ________

10. Did a household member go to prison?

    Yes No If yes enter 1 _______

Now add up your "Yes" answers: _______ This is your ACE Score.

The results of the survey—which is administered to adults only, not children—can be an important beginning point for discussion about the ways that trauma manifests. The ACE-Q can also be used to open up dialogue about how current behavior may be linked to childhood experiences and can assist individuals in understanding the impact of childhood adversity. Another benefit is that the client will know they are not alone in these experiences, paving the way for greater self-awareness and coping skills. In all of these ways, the survey can contribute to the healing process for survivors of ACEs.

Summary

Adult children of dysfunctional family homes are left with fundamental problems in basic trust, autonomy, and initiative. Even among dysfunctional family homes, there is a great deal of variability in how often dysfunctional interactions and behaviors occur and in the kinds and the severity of their dysfunction. An insidious part of complex trauma is that it usually begins in the home and a vast majority of those responsible for child maltreatment are the children's own parent(s) in the context of a dysfunctional family unit. When the person who is meant to protect you and care for you is also the one that harms you, this creates a significant internal conflict. Winnicott (1990) proposed that effective parenting had to come from a place of love. This optimum parental love involves surrendering of the ego and putting aside one's own needs for the sake of close, intensive listening to another person whose unique otherness is respected and sought to be understood (1990). Adaptation to the child's world and attunement to their needs must come from a place of surrender of one's own needs, so as not to oppress the child's sense of self (Winnicott, 1990). This also relates to the trust-building component of the clinical relationship. The subsequent chapter shall explore the role of dissociation and affect regulation in the treatment of C-PTSD.

Questions and Activities for Discussion and Further Reflection

1. What are the core differences between clear communication and communication deviance?
2. Do you understand the terms (i) enmeshment, (ii) triangulation, and (iii) pathological accommodation?
3. What are the implications of a client role within a dysfunctional family system on the clinical relationship? (What would be the challenges to treating the hero, the scapegoat, etc.?)
4. How would you revise the ACE-Q to reflect the childhood experience of racism, discrimination, and displacement?

Exercise

1. Class Discussion Prompt: Reflect on the glossary of terms provided in this chapter, have you experienced communication deviance directly? Have you encountered any of the examples of communication deviance professionally. If there is a term that you are aware of that is not included on the list please contact the author directly.
2. Self-administer the ACE privately. Any personal reflections on the questionnaire can be journaled reflectively.

References

Aponte, H. J., & Van Deusen, J. M. (1981). Structural family therapy. In A. S. Gurman & D. P. Kniskem (Eds.), *Handbook of family therapy* (pp. 310–361). New York, NY: Brunner Mazel Inc.

Baker, J. D., & Williamson, D. A. (1989). Psychological profiles of adult children of alcoholics in search of therapy. *Counselling Psychology Quarterly, 2*, 451–457.

Bateson, G., Jackson, D. D., Haley, J., & Weakland, J. (1963). A note on the double bind – 1962. *Family Process, 2*, 154–161.

Black, C. (1981). *It will never happen to me*. Denver, CO: M.A.C.

Bowen, M. (1976). Theory in the practice of psychotherapy. In P. Guerin (Ed.), *Family therapy: Theory and practice* (pp. 42–90). New York, NY: Gardner.

Brandchaft, B. (2007). Systems of pathological accommodation and change in analysis. *Psychoanalytic Psychology, 24*, 667–687. https://doi.org/10.1037/0736-9735.24.4.667

Brown, D. W., Anda, R. F., Felitti, V. J., Edwards, V. J., Malarcher, A. M., Croft, J. B., & Giles, W. H. (2010). Adverse childhood experiences are associated with the risk of lung cancer: A prospective cohort study. *BMC Public Health, 10*, 20. https://doi.org/10.1186/1471-2458-10-20

Buelow, G. (1994). Treatment of role stereotypy in severally dysfunctional and chemically dependent families. *Journal of Child and Adolescent Substance Abuse, 3*, 13–24.

Centers for Disease Control and Prevention. (n.d.). *Major findings ACE study*. Division of Adult and Community Health, National Center for Chronic Disease Prevention and Health Promotion.

Centers for Disease Control and Prevention, National Center for Injury Prevention and Control, Division of Violence Prevention. (2014, May). *The Adverse Childhood Experiences (ACE) Study. cdc.gov*. Atlanta, Georgia. Archived from the original on 27 December 2015. https://www.cdc.gov/violenceprevention/acestudy/index.html

Derefinko, K. J., Salgado García, F. I., Talley, K. M., Bursac, Z., Johnson, K. C., Murphy, J. G., … Sumrok, D. D. (2019). Adverse childhood experiences predict opioid relapse during treatment among rural adults. *Addictive Behaviors, 96*, 171–174. https://doi.org/10.1016/j.addbeh.2019.05.008

Ditton, P., Green, R. J., & Singer, M. T. (1987). Communication deviance: A comparison between parents of learning disabled and normally achieving students. *Family Process, 26*, 75–87.

Doctors, S. R. (2017). Brandchafts's pathological accommodation – What it is and what it isn't. *Psychoanalysis, Self and Context, 12*, 45–59. https://doi.org/10.1080/15551024.2017.1251184

Felitti, V. J., Anda, R. F., Nordenberg, D., Williamson, D. F., Spitz, A. M., Edwards, V., … Marks, J. S. (1998). Relationship of childhood abuse and household dysfunction to many of the leading causes of death in adults. The adverse childhood experiences (ACE) study. *American Journal of Preventive Medicine, 14*, 245–258.

Fisher, G. L., Jenkins, S. J., Harrison, T. C., & Jesch, K. (1993). Personality characteristics of ACOAs, other adults from dysfunctional families and adults of nondysfunctional families. *International Journal of the Addictions, 28*, 477–485.

Harrington, C. M., & Metzler, A. E. (1997). Are adult children of dysfunctional families with alcoholism different from adult children of dysfunctional families without alcoholism? A look at committed, intimate relationships. *Journal of Counseling Psychology, 44*(1), 102–107. Retrieved from http://proxy.library.nyu.edu/login?url=https://search-proquest-com.proxy.library.nyu.edu/docview/57532088?accountid=12768

Herman, J. L. (1992). *Trauma and recovery: The aftermath of violence*. New York, NY: Basic Books.

Hinz, L. D. (1990). College student adult children of alcoholics: Psychological resilience or emotional distance? *Journal of Substance Abuse, 2*, 449–457.

Jenkins, S. J., Fisher, G. L., & Harrison, T. C. (1993). Adult children of dysfunctional families: Childhood roles. *Journal of Mental Health Counselling, 15*, 310–319.

Klein, M. (1946). Notes on some schizoid mechanisms. In R. Money-Kyrle (Ed.), *The writings of Melanie Klein* (Vol. 3, pp. 1–24). London, UK: The Hogarth Press.

McKenna, T., & Pickens, R. (1983). Personality characteristics of alcoholic children of alcoholics. *Journal of Studies on Alcohol, 44*, 688–700.

O'Shea Brown, G. (2020a). The impact of anomie and societal splitting on the self: Suicide among members of the travelling Community of Ireland. *Journal of PsychoHistory, 48*(2).

O'Shea Brown, G. (2020b). Internal family systems informed eye movement desensitization and reprocessing: An integrative technique for treatment of complex posttraumatic stress disorder. *International Body Psychotherapy Journal, 19*(2).

O'Shea Brown, G. (2021). Reflections on providing virtual eye movement desensitization and reprocessing therapy in the wake of COVID-19: Survival through adaptation. In C. Tosone (Ed.), *Shared trauma, shared resilience during a pandemic: Social work in the time of COVID-19*. Cham, Switzerland: Springer.

Riggs, D. W., & Bartholomaeus, C. (2018). Gaslighting in the context of clinical interactions with parents of transgender children. *Sexual and Relationship Therapy, 33*(4), 382-394. http://dx.doi.org.proxy.library.nyu.edu/10.1080/14681994.2018.1444274

Rosengren, K. S., Behrend, D. A., & Perlmutter, M. (1993). Parental influences on children's cognition. In R. Pasnak & M. L. Howe (Eds.), *Emerging themes in cognitive development, volume 2: Competencies* (pp. 103–124). London, UK: Springer-Verlag.

Singer, M. T., Wynne, M. D., & Toohey, M. L. (1978). Communication disorders and the families of schizophrenics. In L. C. Wynne, R. L. Cromwell, & S. Matthyse (Eds.), *The nature of schizophrenia* (pp. 499–511). New York, NY: John Wiley.

Webb, W., Post, P., Robinson, B., & Moreland, L. (1992). Self-concept, anxiety, and knowledge exhibited by adult children of alcoholics and adult children of nonalcoholics. *Journal of Alcohol and Drug Education, 38*, 106–114.

Wegscheider, S. (1981). *Another chance: Hope and health for the alcoholic family*. Palo Alto, CA: Science and Behavior Books.

Williams, L. M., & Hiebert, W. J. (2001). Challenging the belief system behind enmeshment. *Journal of Clinical Activities, Assignments & Handouts in Psychotherapy Practice, 1*(2), 17–28. Retrieved from http://proxy.library.nyu.edu/login?url=https://search-proquest-com.proxy.library.nyu.edu/docview/61466109?accountid=12768

Winnicott, D. W. (1990). *Home is where we start from – Essays of a psychoanalyst*. New York, NY: W.W. Norton & Co. Inc.

Zarse, E. M., Neff, M. R., Yoder, R., Hulvershorn, L., Chambers, J. E., & Chambers, R. A. (2019). The adverse childhood experiences questionnaire: Two decades of research on childhood trauma as a primary cause of adult mental illness, addiction, and medical diseases. *Cogent Medicine, 6*(1), 1581447. https://doi-org.proxy.library.nyu.edu/10.1080/2331205x.2019.1581447

Chapter 5
Dissociation

Dissociation is a state in which certain thoughts, emotions, sensations, and/or memories are compartmentalized, resulting in discontinuities in conscious awareness (Forgash & Copeley, 2008; van der Hart, Nijenhuis, & Steele, 2006). Trauma survivors often present as fragmented in their sense of self (Janet, 1889; Siegel, 1999). Janet (1889) describes dissociation as a mental structure in which traumatic and stressful life events are excluded from conscious awareness. Dissociation is a natural part of trauma and allows the individual to survive in a precarious environment through the use of cognitive dissonance (Siegel, 1999; van der Hart et al., 2006). This disruption of normal integration has many adaptive advantages, as well as pathological consequences. From an adaptive standpoint, dissociation refers to a compartmentalization of experience: elements of an experience are not integrated into a unitary whole but are stored in isolated fragments (O'Shea Brown, 2020). Thus, dissociation can be thought of as a way of organizing information (van der Hart et al., 2006; van der Hart, van der Kolk, & Boon, 1998).

Another way to conceptualize dissociation is as a fog that emerges to shroud certain parts of experiences that are too overwhelming and painful to be faced fully. The sensory experience of the traumatic event may be split off from other aspects of the experience and recalled later in a fragmented way. For instance, a survivor of 9/11 may distinctly remember the smell of burnt rubber, but may report that many aspects or parts of the day feel blurred. Dissociation is at the very heart of trauma; consequently, it is necessary as part of trauma-informed care to understand its causes and symptom presentation, in addition to its clinical significance in the context of complex trauma treatment. This chapter will provide a description of the role, purpose, and function of dissociation from a trauma-informed perspective. The chapter will then explore how dissociative experiencing can be measured in a clinical setting, utilizing the Scale of Dissociative Experiences II. Following an overview of the clinical tool, this chapter will explore the signs and symptoms of dissociation before considering the practice implications of working with

G. O'Shea Brown, *Healing Complex Posttraumatic Stress Disorder*, Essential Clinical Social Work Series, https://doi.org/10.1007/978-3-030-61416-4_5

dissociative clients. Finally, strategies to orient a client to conscious awareness will be explored and illustrated via clinical vignette.

Understanding Dissociation

Dissociation has been described as one of a constellation of symptoms experienced by some survivors of complex trauma as a result of physical abuse, emotional abuse, sexual abuse, or neglect. Though symptoms of dissociation are common in many disorders, such as posttraumatic stress disorder and acute stress disorder, this chapter will focus on dissociation as a common sequela of complex trauma. The *Diagnostic and Statistical Manual of Mental Disorders, 5th Edition* (DSM-5) specifies that dissociation is a disruption to the usually integrated functions of consciousness, memory, identity, or perception of the environment (American Psychiatric Association, 2013). Dissociation can be seen as a continuum which includes a wide array of experiences, from mild detachment from immediate surroundings to more severe detachment from physical and emotional experiences. Notably, it involves detachment from reality rather than a loss of reality, as characterizes psychosis (Cronin, Brand, & Mattanah, 2014; van der Kolk, 2015).

At the more severe end of the spectrum, dissociation can lead to multiple identities. Dissociative identity disorder (DID), previously known as multiple personality disorder, is a complex, posttraumatic developmental disorder (APA, 2013; Putnam, 1997). Studies indicate that dissociative symptoms and a history of severe childhood trauma are present long before DID is suspected or diagnosed (Lewis, Yeager, Swica, Pincus, & Lewis, 1997; Swica, Lewis, & Lewis, 1996). DID causes an individual to develop two or more personalities, configured as a host identity and alter identities. The identities can vary in terms of age, gender, personality characteristics, and history and may even go by unique names. There is often a sense of amnesia among the identities; at times the individual afflicted with DID will have identities that they are unaware of, and at times they are in a state of co-consciousness with an alter (Butcher, Mineka, & Hooley, 2014). The *Diagnostic and Statistical Manual of Mental Disorders, 5th Edition* (DSM-5) (2013) provides the following diagnostic criteria for DID:

> a disruption of identity characterized by two or more distinct personality states. The disruption in identity involves marked discontinuity in sense of self and sense of agency, accompanied by related alterations in affect, behavior, consciousness, memory, perception, cognition, and/or sensory-motor functioning. Recurrent gaps in the recall of everyday events, important personal information, and/or traumatic events that are inconsistent with ordinary forgetting. The symptoms cause clinically significant distress or impairment in social and occupational functioning. (APA, 2013, p.663)

The taboo nature of DID means that this disorder is frequently perceived by the sufferer as shameful and thus hidden, meaning individuals often suffer in silence while painfully aware of their dissociation and complex identity. Research has found that approximately 1% of the general population lives with DID (Brand et al.,

2016; International Society for the Study of Trauma and Dissociation, 2011). Scroppo, Drob, Weinberger, and Eagle (1998) conducted a study with 42 female subjects recruited from outpatient mental health settings and physician referrals. The subjects were divided into 2 subcategories, each comprised of 21 members; by design, one of these groups representing half the total subjects had a DID diagnosis, and the other group, with non-dissociative disorders, served as the control group. The study authors conducted the following assessments prior to recruiting the subjects: a screening process (ensuring each subject was actively engaged in psychotherapy); face-to-face assessment; completion of the Tellegen Absorption Scale Brief Symptom Inventory, Scale of Dissociative Experiences, and Childhood Trauma Questionnaire; and a diagnostic interview using the Dissociative Disorders Interview Schedule. Analysis of the results demonstrated that the DID group showed a distinguishing set of clinical features including a prevalence of childhood trauma, insecure attachment patterns, and a high score in the Scale of Dissociative Experiences compared to the control group. Maldonado and Spiegel (2007) also found high rates of comorbidity among DID and depressive disorders, posttraumatic stress disorder, substance use disorders, and borderline personality disorder. These findings point to how complex and nuanced the treatment and diagnosis of DID must be. The ultimate goal of treatment is to establish integrated functioning of the alter identities and the host identity, preferably through guiding the client in gentle exploration in the context of therapy (Butcher et al., 2014).

Schielke, Brand, and Marsic (2017) conducted a research study with 177 subjects, each paired with a clinician for individual therapy over the course of 30 months. In order to assess the therapeutic change in patients, Schielke et al. (2017) aimed to provide psychometric data for both the patient and the clinician with a clear measure of therapeutic progress of DID patients by administering the "Progress in Treatment Questionnaire – Therapist" (PITQ-t; a therapist report measure) and the "Progress in Treatment Questionnaire – Patient" (PITQ-p; a patient self-report measure). This assessment reviewed the following areas: the quality of the therapeutic relationship; establishing safety; processing trauma; affect and emotional regulation; capacity for developing adaptive coping strategies; management of symptoms; need for external support; and presence of phenomena related to dissociative identities (Schielke et al., 2017). Upon completion of the study, the authors found that the PITQ-t and PITQ-p "demonstrated good internal consistency and evidence of moderate convergent validity in relation to established measures of emotional dysregulation, dissociation, posttraumatic stress disorder, and psychological quality of life, which are characteristic difficulties for DID patients" (Schielke et al., 2017, p.58). This study demonstrated that regular therapy and a strong rapport can greatly benefit the client in developing adaptive strategies to counteract the symptoms of DID. Furthermore, therapeutic interventions and close assessment were both found to be beneficial in fostering emotional regulation, strengthening social relations, and establishing a reduction in self-harm and high-risk behaviors. Most importantly, the study illustrated how patient self-reports providing their assessment of therapy are useful in helping clinicians move forward with a person-centered, ethical treatment approach empowering the client to regain a sense of agency in their treatment plan.

Dissociative phenomena are not confined to individuals living with DID. Research indicates that some level of dissociative experiencing is often present and is a core element within emotional disorders originating from stressful or traumatic life events (Brand et al., 2016; O'Shea Brown, 2020; van der Hart et al., 2006). At the milder end of the spectrum, dissociation can be seen as a coping mechanism or defense mechanism enabling an individual to minimize or tolerate stress, and symptom presentation can be at times difficult to identify (van der Hart, van der Kolk, & Boon, 1998). Dissociative experiences can be categorized into unique categories including dissociative amnesia, depersonalization, and derealization.

Dissociative Amnesia refers to the inability to recall important personal information, usually of a traumatic or stressful nature (APA, 2013). This can often present in the context of episodes of self-harming behavior, violence, or suicide attempts. A client may say, *I had a terrible day and thought about self-harming all day long. I attempted to counteract these feelings by having a warm bath, but everything after that is foggy…I woke up in a cold bath with lesions all over my thighs. I don't remember cutting myself with the razor but it must have happened.*

Depersonalization refers to the persistent or recurrent feeling of being detached from one's own mental process or body, but is accompanied by intact reality testing, e.g., a client may describe dreamlike state, unreality of self or body, or slowed time perception (APA, 2013). Symptoms of depersonalization may include but are not restricted to feeling numb (emotionally or physically); feelings that you are an outside observer of your thoughts, feelings, or body; feeling not in control of your speech or movements; or a sense that your memories lack emotion. Depersonalization may occur while recalling a traumatic life event or even during a challenging session. The client may have the sensation of watching themselves from an out-of-body vantage point, as if they were seeing themselves in the third person. This has a way of titrating the experience, as if the trauma was happening to someone else and not to them directly. A client may say, *I see myself being molested by my uncle, but not through my eyes. It is as if it were happening to someone else. I see him leaning over her; he is fat, disgusting, and smells of vodka. She is looking at the ceiling trying to pretend to be somewhere else. I am looking down at a 45-degree angle from above.*

Derealization refers to persistent or recurrent instances of unreality of surroundings, with the world experienced as unreal, dreamlike, or distorted (APA, 2013). Symptoms of derealization may include feelings of being alienated from or unfamiliar with your surroundings, as if living in a movie or a dream; feeling emotionally disconnected from people you care about; surroundings appearing distorted, blurry, colorless, two-dimensional, or artificial; or a heightened awareness and clarity of your surroundings. Other signs of derealization include distortions in perception of time, such as recent events feeling like distant past, and distortions of distance and the size and shape of objects. A client may say, *I walked in on my wife having* *sex with my friend. I thought I was hallucinating. It seemed bizarre and unreal to me. It felt not real – it was like a weird dream!*

Depersonalization and derealization can cause significant impairment in social and occupational functioning. The above dissociative experiences are not caused by the physiological effects of an ingested substance or a medical condition. Measuring for dissociation at the beginning of clinical treatment can help the clinician to ascertain where the client is on the continuum of dissociative experiencing. In addition, the clinician is able to better understand the client's perception of reality.

Measuring Dissociation

The Scale of Dissociative Experiences II (DESII), created by Carlson and Putnam (1993), is a psychological self-assessment questionnaire that measures dissociative symptoms in adults. (Adolescents and children should be administered different age-appropriate versions.) The DESII measures a wide variety of types of dissociation, including both problematic dissociative experiences and normal dissociative experiences (e.g., day-dreaming). It is used as a screening tool for a variety of dissociative disorders. For example, the diagnostic symptom criteria of PTSD includes non-fear-based symptoms, such as risky or destructive behavior, overly negative self-concept, exaggerated blame of self or others for causing the trauma, negative affect, decreased interest in activities, and feelings of isolation (APA, 2013), but criteria also include dissociative symptoms such as depersonalization and derealization. Individuals with a diagnosis of C-PTSD or PTSD will therefore score highly in the DESII. However dissociative symptoms are not included in the diagnostic criteria of acute stress disorder. The DESII asks questions which are designed to gather information about experiences that you may have in your daily life. It is important to know that the frequency of the experiences is highly significant. Furthermore, experiences are negated if they occur when under the influence of alcohol, substances, or drugs. There are 28 questions. When answering the questions, the recipient is asked to determine to what degree each experience described in the question applies to them and then select the number to show what percentage of the time they have had the experience. For example, 0% indicates never, 20–30% indicates sometimes (less than half the time), and 100% indicates always. The scale is shown in Fig. 5.1.

The DESII was designed to measure the frequency of dissociative experiences. Per the above answer key, when scoring the DESII, some questions relate to "Amnesia Factor" (memory loss), "Depersonalization/Derealization Factor" (detachment from the mind/body or a sense of unreality), and "Absorption Factor" (becoming so distracted by an activity that you are unaware of the world around you). When scoring this questionnaire, it is important to note that you must drop the 0 on the percentage, for example, 40% becomes 4 and 50% becomes 5. After scoring the chart, it can be helpful to explore and learn more about the experiences of

DES

Eve Bernstein Carlson, PhD & Frank W. Putnam, MD

Directions: This questionnaire consists of twenty-eight questions about experiences that you may have in your daily life. We are interested in how often you have these experiences. It is important, however, that your answers show how often these experiences happen to you when you **are not** under the influence of alcohol or drugs. To answer the questions, please determine to what degree the experience described in the question applies to you and circle the number to show what percentage of the time you have the experience.

Example:

0% (never) 10 20 30 40 50 60 70 80 90 100% (always)

Date________________ **Age** ____________ **Sex: M F**

1. Some people have the experience of driving or riding in a car or bus or subway and suddenly realizing that they don't remember what has happened during all or pan of the trip. Circle a number to show what percentage of the time this happens to you.
0% 10 20 30 40 50 60 70 80 90 100%

2. Some people find that sometimes they are listening to someone talk and they suddenly realize that they did not hear part or all of what was said. Circle a number to show what percentage of the time this happens to you.
0% 10 20 30 40 50 60 70 80 90 100%

3. Some people have the experience of finding themselves in a place and having no idea how they got there. Circle a number to show what percentage of the time this happens to you.
0% 10 20 30 40 50 60 70 80 90 100%

4. Some people have the experience of finding themselves dressed in clothes that they don't remember putting on. Circle a number to show what percentage of the time this happens to you.
0% 10 20 30 40 50 60 70 80 90 100%

5. Some people have the experience of finding new things among their belongings that they do not remember buying. Circle a number to show what percentage of the time this happens to you.
0% 10 20 30 40 50 60 70 80 90 100%

6. Some people sometimes find that they are approached by people who they do not know who call them by another name or insist that they have met them before. Circle a number to show what percentage of the time this happens to you.
0% 10 20 30 40 50 60 70 80 90 100%

7. Some people sometimes have the experience of feeling as though they are standing next to themselves or watching themselves do something and they actually see themselves as if they were looking at another person. Circle a number to show what percentage of the time this happens to you.
0% 10 20 30 40 50 60 70 80 90 100%

8. Some people are told that they sometimes do not recognize friends or family members. Circle a number to show what percentage of the time this happens to you.
0% 10 20 30 40 50 60 70 80 90 100%

9. Some people find that they have no memory for some important events in their lives (for example, a wedding or graduation). Circle a number to show what percentage of the time this happens to you.
0% 10 20 30 40 50 60 70 80 90 100%

10. Some people have the experience of being accused of lying when they do not think that they have lied. Circle a number to show what percentage of the time this happens to you.
0% 10 20 30 40 50 60 70 80 90 100%

11. Some people have the experience of looking in a mirror and not recognizing themselves. Circle a number to show what percentage of the time this happens to you.
0% 10 20 30 40 50 60 70 80 90 100%

12. Some people have the experience of feeling that other people, objects, and the world around them are not real. Circle a number to show what percentage of the time this happens to you.
0% 10 20 30 40 50 60 70 80 90 100%

13. Some people have the experience of feeling that their body does not seem to belong to them. Circle a number to show what percentage of the time this happens to you.
0% 10 20 30 40 50 60 70 80 90 100%

Fig. 5.1 The Scale of Dissociative Experiences, Version II (DESII). (Reprinted from Dissociation, 6(1), Carlson, E. B., & Putnam, F. W., An update on the Dissociative Experiences Scale, Appendix A, 1993, with permission from the International Society for the Study of Trauma and Dissociation)

14. Some people have the experience of sometimes remembering a past event so vividly that they feel as if they were reliving that *event.* Circle a number to show what percentage of the time this happens to you.

0% 10 20 30 40 50 60 70 80 90 100%

15. Some people have the experience of not being sure whether things that they remember happening really did happen or whether they just dreamed them. Circle a number to show what percentage of the time this happens to you.

0% 10 20 30 40 50 60 70 80 90 100%

16. Some people have the experience of being in a familiar place but finding it strange and unfamiliar. Circle a number to show what percentage of the time this happens to you.

0% 10 20 30 40 50 60 70 80 90 100%

17. Some people find that when they are watching television or a movie they become so absorbed in the story that they are unaware of other events happening around them. Circle a number to show what percentage of the time this happens to you.

0% 10 20 30 40 50 60 70 80 90 100%

18. Some people find that they become so involved in a fantasy or daydream that it feels as though it were really happening to them. Circle a number to show what percentage of the time this happens to you.

0% 10 20 30 40 50 60 70 80 90 100%

19. Some people find that they sometimes are able to ignore pain. Circle a number to show what percentage of the time this happens to you.

0% 10 20 30 40 50 60 70 80 90 100%

20. Some people find that they sometimes sit staring off into space, thinking of nothing, and are not aware of the passage of time. Circle a number to show what percentage of the time this happens to you.

0% 10 20 30 40 50 60 70 80 90 100%

21. Some people sometimes find that when they are alone they talk out loud to themselves. Circle a number to show what percentage of the time this happens to you.

0% 10 20 30 40 50 60 70 80 90 100%

22. Some people find that in one situation they may act so differently compared with another situation that they *feel* almost as if they were two different people. Circle a number to show what percentage of the time this happens to you.

0% 10 20 30 40 50 60 70 80 90 100%

23. Some people sometimes find that in certain situations they are able to do things with amazing ease and spontaneity that would usually be difficult for them (for example, sports, work, social situations, etc.). Circle a number to show what percentage of the time this happens to you.

0% 10 20 30 40 50 60 70 80 90 100%

24. Some people sometimes find that they cannot remember whether they have done something or have just thought about doing that thing (for example, not knowing whether they have mailed a letter or have just thought about mailing it). Circle a number to show what percentage of the time this happens to you.

0% 10 20 30 40 50 60 70 80 90 100%

25. Some people find evidence that they have done things that they do not remember doing. Circle a number to show what percentage of the time this happens to you.

0% 10 20 30 40 50 60 70 80 90 100%

26. Some people sometimes find writings, drawings, or notes among their belongings that they must have done but cannot remember doing. Circle a number to show what percentage of the time this happens to you.

0% 10 20 30 40 50 60 70 80 90 100%

27. Some people sometimes find that they hear voices inside their head that tell them to do things or comment on things that they are doing. Circle a number to show what percentage of the time this happens to you.

0% 10 20 30 40 50 60 70 80 90 100%

28. Some people sometimes feel as if they are looking at the world through a fog so that people and objects appear far away or unclear. Circle a number to show what percentage of the time this happens to you.

0% 10 20 30 40 50 60 70 80 90 100%

Fig. 5.1 (continued)

the recipient as a way of understanding their perception of reality. At this point, you can provide psychoeducation and guidance on the role, purpose, and function of dissociation and take time to answer their questions and hear their reflections.

Working with Dissociative Clients

Understanding, diagnosing, and treating dissociation can be challenging. Relatively few clinicians receive training in accurately diagnosing and treating DID, despite the existence of expert consensus guidelines and treatment recommendations (Brand, Lanius, Loewenstein, Vermetten, & Spiegel, 2012; Brand, Myrick, et al., 2012; ISSTD, 2011). In the context of treating complex trauma, you are highly likely to encounter trauma survivors with dissociative symptoms. We must remember that it is rare that clients with a history of childhood trauma do not have at least some dissociative symptoms (Brand, Lanius, et al., 2012; Brand, Myrick, et al., 2012; ISSTD, 2011). Symptoms of fragmentation, depersonalization, self-hypnosis, out-of-body experiences, and internal conflict between ego states can emerge following a trauma. In evaluating an individual's adaptive versus maladaptive uses of dissociation, it can be helpful as with the treatment of complex trauma for treatment to be a trauma-informed, multimodal, and multi-phased (O'Shea Brown, 2020). Effective techniques such as somatic-based therapies, ego state work, and internal family systems will be discussed in-depth in Chaps. 8 and 9.

The ultimate goal of treatment of dissociation is to establish integrated functioning of the self and the body, preferably through guiding the client in gentle exploration in the context of therapy (O'Shea Brown, 2020). This can be achieved by supporting the client in stabilizing symptoms related to dissociation and PTSD with the provision of psychoeducation and the application of stabilization and grounding techniques (Brand, Lanius, et al., 2012; Brand, Myrick, et al., 2012; ISSTD, 2011). The purpose of this approach is to decrease self-destructive behaviors, develop awareness and cooperation with dissociated self-states, enhance affect awareness, and develop tolerance of positive affective state (O'Shea Brown, 2020). The therapeutic alliance between the clinician and the client is vitally important for helping clients develop self-awareness and tolerance of affect regulation (Brand et al., 2013; Cronin et al., 2014). To measure a client's ability to tolerate affect regulation, they are thought grounding techniques and encouraged to use them independently as they become more familiar with the sensation of relaxation and other positive feeling states (discussed more in-depth in Chap. 6).

When an individual is experiencing dissociation, they momentarily disconnect from their surroundings, which can stop the traumatic memories in addition to reducing feelings of fear, anxiety, and shame. Remembering the more adaptive uses of dissociation will prevent the pathologizing of dissociative symptoms and remind the client that with the support of therapeutic care, they can turn maladaptive symptoms into adaptive capabilities. Ultimately the trauma survivor is guided toward seeing their body as their partner in survival and healing. Dissociative experiencing can occur during the trauma or later on, when thinking about or being reminded of the trauma. Sometimes dissociation can feel intrusive for the individual. The unmetabolized trauma memories, much like a "skipping disc," may replay the most distressing part of the memory, causing intrusive thoughts, flashbacks, or even numbing. During treatment history, there can be early indicators that a client is experiencing dissociation. For instance, clients with multiple diagnoses and various mental health providers with a poor level of progress or clarity may be suspected of increased dissociative experiencing (Putnam, 1991). Likewise, a client who struggles internally with alternating idealization and devaluation or approach-avoidance of their clinicians, or those who had therapeutic alliances that ended in some unusually dramatic ways, should raise our suspicion (Fisher, 2017). Therefore, during treatment planning, it is important to be open and curious about past experiences of mental health history and therapeutic experiences. In a clinical setting, there are several cues that could indicate a client is experiencing dissociation. Symptoms seen in conjunction with dissociation may include:

- Eye movements [either constant rapid scanning (saccadic) or eye blinking or drooping].
- Eye contact (the client appears to be looking through you or presents with mouth open and eyes glazed over).
- Reported high pain tolerance.
- Change in body temperature, numbness, and tingling.
- Change in body language more typical for young child (in alignment with regressed language or cognition).
- The client may be watching themselves from an outer body experience (depersonalization).
- Reports non-responsiveness to psychopharmacological medications.
- Clients who become mute and cannot be facilitated to verbalize what they are thinking or feeling.
- Client is acting differently than is usual to their baseline presentation, for instance, using a different tone of voice, cadence, different accent, or different gestures.
- Client reports "blackouts" or "loss of time." For instance, a client may say, *I walked 40 blocks in the wrong direction without even noticing.*
- Client is not fully oriented to the present moment. This is evident in trail of thought, focus, and ability to hear you. Client may say, *I just zoned out; What was I just saying; I am sorry—I went somewhere else for a while; I feel the same way I did at the time (of the trauma); I feel numb.*
- (The clinician) feels any of the above on a regular basis when in the room with a specific client. Pay attention to your countertransference.

If you notice any of the above, you can ask the client: "What percentage of you is in the room right now?" If the answer is below 70%, you can begin by asking the client to name three things they can see (that are flat, colorful, soft, etc.), that they can hear, and/or that they can feel. Alternatively, you can invite the client to walk around the room and ask them to examine if a plant is real or fake. This can entice the client to connect with texture, temperature, and scent. You can ask them to choose an object from your bookshelf, perhaps an ornate candle – then, with focused attention, they can describe the scent, the color, and the décor. Alternatively, you can ask them to notice their toes in their shoes and their seat on their chair and to touch each finger individually with their thumb, verbally guiding them in a soft but anchoring voice. Following this technique, you can once again ask, "What percentage of you is in the room?" If the above simple techniques do not orient the client back to into present moment, as evidenced by a reported percentage of 70% or more, you can offer another resource. You may suggest a grounding technique to bring them back to the present moment or as a means to bring them back into their body. The intention behind this grounding exercise is to assist the client in recognizing the signs and symptoms of their dissociation and to teach them the skills to independently manage symptoms so that these symptoms do not adversely impact their life in the present moment (O'Shea Brown, 2021). The above grounding techniques are intended to bring the client back into present awareness. The client is learning to differentiate the past from the present moment and also learning about their somatic awareness (ability to be in their body). Grounding techniques are helpful for orienting a client into the present moment when dissociation arises and also may work as a remedy for stress triggers.

Clinical Vignette

Valentina[1] is a 39-year-old, single Hispanic female employed full-time as a social services director. She recently escaped a domestically abusive relationship. She endured years of emotional, physical, and sexual abuse. During session, she at times will present with the following dissociative symptoms: unexpected lapses in attention, momentary avoidance of eye contact with no memory, and staring into space for several moments while appearing to be in a daze. This often occurs when she speaks about her experiences of the relationship. The following is a grounding technique adapted from Elan Shapiro's "the four elements" technique (Shapiro, 2012). The following excerpt illustrates the process of Valentina being guided through the steps of a grounding technique while engaging in guided breath work.

Clinician: Valentina, I think I lost you for a little while, where did you go?

Valentina: I don't know, what was I saying…my mind just went blank. That is all.

Clinician: I think that the protective fog came in when you were accessing some painful material. How would you feel about taking a few moments to do a grounding exercise?

Valentina: Yes, that would be nice – I am sorry.

Clinician: Valentina, do not apologize, just know that your body and your mind are hard-wired to protect you. Sometimes memories are too painful to hold, so

[1] A pseudonym has been used to preserve confidentiality.

you experience the protective fog. I would like to teach you a technique to use whenever you feel like you are drifting away.

Valentina: That makes me feel more normal. You're right – maybe it protects me from the pain of remembering.

Clinician: Yes, a protective reflex to pain...Take three deep breaths.... sit back in the chair, connect with your body, and begin to breathe deep into the stomach. Breathe in through the nose with long generous exhales through birthday-candle lips.

Valentina: (body language becomes more expansive; eyes are closed and jaw is unclenched).

Clinician: You are seated with your feet on the ground (Pause).

Valentina: (nods). (Shoulders drop, jaw is unclenched, client has a slight grin).

Clinician: We are now going to do a grounding exercise– in this exercise, we will explore the four elements: earth, air, water, and fire.

The first element is earth.

Take a minute or two to 'land' in to the body and surrender to gravity… to be here now.

Place both feet on the ground, feel the chair supporting you.

As you continue feeling the security of your feet on the ground, you feel centered as you breathe in and out.

Valentina: (breath deepens, feet planted firmly on the ground).

Clinician: The next element is air. As you continue feeling the security of your feet on the ground, take three or four deeper, slower breaths from your stomach, making sure to breathe all the way out to make room for fresh, energizing air.

You may even begin to notice the temperature of the room and the sound of your breathing.

As you breathe out, imagine that you are letting go of some of the stress, breathing it out. As you breathe in, focus inwards to your center.

Valentina: (nods). Eyes are closed, no signs of tension on the face, jaw appears unclenched.

Clinician: The next element I want you to bring your awareness to is water.

Notice if you have saliva in your mouth.

Perhaps you can make more saliva… If you are able to do so let me know by nodding.

Valentina: (nods)

Clinician: Wonderful. When you are anxious or stressed, your mouth often dries, since part of the stress emergency response (which has to do with the sympathetic nervous system) is to shut off the digestive system.

However, when you are able to create saliva, this is your body's way of knowing you are in a state of rest and repair.

When you salivate, you switch on the digestive system again.

This is the reason why people are offered water or tea after a difficult experience.

When you make saliva, your mind can optimally control your thoughts and your body. Direct your attention to making saliva in your mouth, knowing you are now in a state of rest and repair.

Valentina: (Gentle swishing in her mouth.)

Clinician: As you continue feeling the security of your feet on the ground. Take a moment to connect with the elements of earth, air and water.

You feel centered as you breathe in and out, and feel calm and in control as you produce more and more saliva. Direct your attention to feeling good in your body.

Valentina: (Swishing, deep diaphragmatic breathing).

Clinician: As you continue feeling the security now of your feet on the ground, and feel centered as you breathe in and out, and feel calm and in control as you produce more and more saliva, notice how you feel in your body.

Valentina: I am safe and strong.

Clinician: As you connect with the elements of earth, air and water – continue to breathe and be here now. I want you to imagine a benevolent Olympian torch lighting your way forward. As you allow the fire to light your path, bring to mind an experience of a place where you feel calm.

Valentina: I am at a house David[2] *and I sometimes visit by the beach. I am sitting on the back deck. I have just practiced yoga. I can smell the ocean in the distance. It's a warm day. I feel Zen.*

Clinician: Notice the light, colors, smells, and sounds. Where do you feel it in your body?

Valentina: I feel a lightness washing over me, as if my tension has been soothed away. I smell the ocean air. My shoulders feel soft and my stomach feel calm.

Clinician: Allow that feeling to spread and flow throughout your body and breath.

Valentina: (Breathes deeply).

Clinician: (after a long pause). When you are ready, I want you to take three deep breaths, begin to notice your feet on the ground, your tongue in your mouth and the temperature of this room as you slowly, slowly reenter this room by opening your eyes.

Valentina: (opens eyes) I am back.

In this clinical vignette, Valentina becomes dissociative while accessing painful material from her past. In order to bring her back into her body and orient her to the present, she is guided through a grounding technique. There is also some light psychoeducation intended to depathologize her experiences of dissociation, as it is referred to as "a protective fog." A central feature of complex trauma is a loss of the ability to physiologically modulate stress responses, in addition to a diminished capacity to utilize bodily signals (van der Kolk, McFarlane, & Weisaeth, 1996). This

[2] A pseudonym has been used to preserve confidentiality.

can lead to heightened symptoms of emotional reactivity or dissociative experiencing. Grounding techniques can be very effective in increasing affect tolerance when used to enhance mindfulness or the ability to notice a feeling or bodily sensation and accompanying emotions.

Summary

Dissociation can be thought of as a fog that emerges to shroud certain parts of experiences that are too overwhelming and painful to be faced fully. The sensory experience of the traumatic event may be split off from other aspects of the experience and recalled later in a fragmented way. For instance, a survivor of 9/11 may distinctly remember the smell of burnt rubber, but may report that many aspects or parts of the day feel blurred. Dissociation is at the very heart of trauma; consequently, in trauma-informed care, it is necessary to understand its causes and symptom presentation, in addition to its clinical significance in the context of complex trauma treatment. It is critical for clinicians to build strong attunement and communication skills to ensure optimal connection with the client during dissociation, in addition to providing non-pathologizing psychoeducation and grounding techniques to empower the client to manage their symptoms outside of the therapy room.

Questions and Activities for Discussion and Further Reflection

1. What are the core differences between mild and severe dissociation?
2. Do you understand the terms (i) derealization and (ii) depersonalization?

Exercise

1. Print out the DESII screening tool.
2. Self-administer this clinical tool and reflect on your experience of dissociative experiencing.
3. Class discussion in groups of 2–4 addressing one of the following:
   - How does dissociation promote survival?
   - What are your thoughts on how dissociation is reflected in pop culture, and how does this differ from reality?
   - How would you recognize that a client was dissociative?

References

American Psychiatric Association. (2013). *Diagnostic and statistical manual of mental disorders* (5th ed.). Washington, DC: American Psychiatric Publishing.

Brand, B. L., Lanius, R., Loewenstein, R. J., Vermetten, E., & Spiegel, D. (2012). Where are we going? An update on assessment, treatment, and neurobiological research in dissociative disorders as we move towards the DSM-5. *Journal of Trauma & Dissociation, 13*, 931.

Brand, B. L., McNary, S. W., Myrick, A. C., Loewenstein, R. J., Classen, C. C., Lanius, R. A., et al. (2013). A longitudinal, naturalistic study of dissociative disorder patients treated by community clinicians. *Psychological Trauma: Theory, Research, Practice, & Policy, 5*(4), 301308.

Brand, B. L., Myrick, A. C., Loewenstein, R. J., Classen, C. C., Lanius, R., McNary, S. W., et al. (2012). A survey of practices and recommended treatment interventions among expert therapists treating patients with dissociative identity disorder and dissociative disorder not otherwise specified. *Psychological Trauma: Theory, Research, Practice, and Policy, 4*(5), 490500.

Brand, B. L., Sar, V., Stavropoulos, P., Krüger, C., Korzekwa, M., Martínez-Taboas, A., & Middleton, W. (2016). Separating fact from fiction: An empirical examination of six myths about dissociative identity disorder. *Harvard Review of Psychiatry, 24*(4), 257–270.

Butcher, J. N., Mineka, S., & Hooley, J. M. (2014). *Abnormal psychology* (15th ed.). Boston, MA: Prentice Hall.

Carlson, E. B., & Putnam, F. W. (1993). An update on the dissociative experiences scale. *Dissociation, 6*(1), 16–27.

Cronin, E., Brand, B. L., & Mattanah, J. F. (2014). The impact of the therapeutic alliance on treatment outcome in patients with dissociative disorders. *European Journal of Psychotraumatology, 5*. https://doi.org/10.3402/ejpt.v5.22676

Fisher, J. (2017). *Healing the fragmented selves of trauma survivors: Overcoming internal alienation*. New York, NY: Routledge.

Forgash, C., & Copeley, M. (2008). *Healing the heart of trauma and dissociation with EMDR and ego state therapy*. New York, NY: Springer.

International Society for the Study of Trauma and Dissociation. (2011). Guidelines for treating dissociative identity disorder in adults, third revision: Summary version. *Journal of Trauma & Dissociation, 12*(2), 115187.

Janet, P. (1889). *L'Automatisme psychologique*. Paris, France: Felix Alcan. (Reprint: Société Pierre Janet, Paris, 1973).

Lewis, D. O., Yeager, C. A., Swica, Y., Pincus, J. H., & Lewis, M. (1997). Objective documentation of child abuse and dissociation in 12 murderers with dissociative identity disorder. *Am J Psychiatry, 154*, 1703–1710.

Maldonado, J. R., & Spiegel, D. (2007). Dissociative disorders. In J. A. Bourgeois, R. H. Hales, & S. C. Yudofsky (Eds.), *The American Psychiatric Publishing Board prep and review guide for psychiatry* (pp. 251–258). Washington, DC: American Psychiatric Publishing.

O'Shea Brown, G. (2020). Internal family systems informed eye movement desensitization and reprocessing: An integrative technique for treatment of complex posttraumatic stress disorder. *International Body Psychotherapy Journal, 19*(2), 112–122.

O'Shea Brown, G. (2021). Reflections on providing virtual eye movement desensitization and reprocessing therapy in the wake of COVID-19: Survival through adaptation. In C. Tosone (Ed.), *Shared trauma, shared resilience during a pandemic: Social work in the time of COVID-19*. Cham, Switzerland: Springer.

Putnam, F. W. (1991). Dissociative phenomena. In A. Tasman & S. M. Goldfinger (Eds.), *American psychiatric press review of psychiatry* (Vol. 10, pp. 145–160). Washington, DC: American Psychiatric Association.

Putnam, F. W. (1997). *Dissociation in children and adolescents: A developmental perspective*. New York, NY: Guilford.

Schielke, H., Brand, B., & Marsic, A. (2017). Assessing therapeutic change in patients with severe dissociative disorders: The progress in treatment questionnaire, therapist and patient measures.

European Journal of Psychotraumatology, 8(1), 1380471. https://doi.org/10.1080/20008198.2017.1380471

Scroppo, J. C., Drob, S. L., Weinberger, J. L., & Eagle, P. (1998). Identifying dissociative identity disorder: A self-report and projective study. *Journal of Abnormal Psychology, 107*(2), 272–284. https://doi.org/10.1037/0021-843X.107.2.272

Shapiro, E. (2012). 4 Elements exercise. *Journal of EMDR Practice and Research, 1*(2), 113–115.

Siegel, D. J. (1999). *The developing mind: Toward a neurobiology of interpersonal experience*. New York, NY: Guilford Press.

Swica, Y., Lewis, D. O., & Lewis, M. (1996). Child abuse and dissociative identity disorder/multiple personality disorder: The documentation of childhood maltreatment and the corroboration of symptoms. *Child and Adolescent Psychiatric Clinics of North America, 5*, 431–447.

van der Hart, O., Nijenhuis, E., & Steele, K. (2006). *The haunted self: Structural dissociation and the treatment of chronic traumatization*. New York, NY: Norton.

van der Hart, O., van der Kolk, B. A., & Boon, S. (1998). Treatment of dissociative disorders. In J. D. Bremner & C. R. Marmar (Eds.), *Trauma, memory, and dissociation* (Progress in psychiatry, No. 54, pp. 253–283). Washington, DC: American Psychiatric Association.

van der Kolk, B. A. (2015). *The body keeps the score: Brain, mind and body in the healing of trauma*. New York, NY: Viking Press.

van der Kolk, B. A., McFarlane, A., & Weisaeth, L. (1996). *Traumatic stress*. New York, NY: Guilford Press.

Chapter 6
Trauma and the Body

Unresolved and unexpressed trauma remains dormant in the body, festering and oppressing the trauma survivor long after the threat has passed (Levine, 1997). A central feature of complex trauma is a loss of the ability to physiologically modulate stress responses (van der Kolk, McFarlane, & Weisaeth, 1996). This can compromise the ability to utilize body signals and increase the risk of an immune system impairment, which has been found to lead to stress-related illnesses (Lowenstein & Goodwin, 1999). It has been established that exposure to the threat of trauma stimulates the autonomic nervous system, resulting in sympathetic hyperarousal and parasympathetic hypoarousal states accompanying survival responses such as fight, flight, submission, and freeze (LeDoux, 2002; Ogden, Minton, & Pain, 2006; Porges, 2003; van der Kolk, 1996a, 1996b). For this reason, the treatment of complex trauma should be phase-oriented, multimodal, and skill-focused, with a core emphasis on symptom relief and functional improvement (Briere & Scott, 2006; Courtois, Ford, & Cloitre, 2009).

It is important to note that for many trauma survivors, the body can become a source of pain, intrusion, and shame. Therefore, survivors may often feel disconnected from their bodies. The foundation of trauma healing begins with enhancing the survivor's awareness and knowledge about the body's responses to trauma, with the ultimate goal of locating a sense of safety within the body. This allows the survivor to operate out of deep self-awareness rather than classic conditioning. This chapter begins by providing an overview of how trauma impacts the mind and body. Second, the significance of affective states will be reviewed through the lens of the Modulation Model and Polyvagal Theory. Subsequently, this chapter will explore the concepts of implicit memory and somatization in the context of complex trauma treatment. Finally, this chapter will review the existing relevant literature exploring the relationship between chronic stress and immune system impairment.

G. O'Shea Brown, *Healing Complex Posttraumatic Stress Disorder*, Essential Clinical Social Work Series, https://doi.org/10.1007/978-3-030-61416-4_6

Mind-Body Connection

Professional understanding and treatment of trauma has evolved to more readily acknowledge the growing collection of empirical work establishing the strength of the mind-body connection. The relationship between the mind and the body has been a prominent debate in both classical and contemporary philosophy, often referred to as the mind-body problem: the question of how to parse the relationship between conscious thought processes of the human mind and the brain as part of the body. There are two divergent schools of thought in understanding the mind-body connection: monism and dualism. Monism postulates oneness and singleness, that is, the belief that there is unity in the derivation of all things (Bunge, 1991). The monist perspective of the mind-body relationship is that there is only one unifying reality, essence, or substance through which everything can be explained. In simple terms, the brain and the mind are one. Conversely, the philosopher René Descartes argued that the mind and the body are distinct substances and part of a person's fundamental duality. Dualism sets forth the doctrine that the mind and the body are different and independent of one another (Searle, 2002). Dualism states that there are two essential parts to each individual: the mind and, more substantially, the body. The body is an extension of the "I" in the observable world. Descartes famously encapsulated this notion when he coined the phrase, "I think, therefore I am," which points to the multiple layers of consciousness. The physical experience of sensing stimuli and the emotional experience of being create a unique individual duality that forms the self. Furthermore, the development of qualia through the personal thoughts, individual emotions, and subjective experiences of the self forms the individual's perception (Crane, 1999).

Cartesian dualism asserts that the mind is a non-bodily entity, a soul, or a mental substance that is separate to the physical material that is the body (Crane, 1999). The body and the face are distinct from the character of the mind. The mind-body problem can demonstrate a misalignment, an existential part of being human (Crane, 1999; Searle, 2002). Both entities are unique and different, but intertwined not out of choice but by force (Chessick, 2009; Gerdes, Segal, & Harmon, 2013). From a dualist perspective, the mind-body problem arises when the two entities are considered separate and come into conflict with one another. This viewpoint considers that the mental substance can exist outside of the body and the body itself does not have the ability to think. The monist perspective of oneness contrasts with the Cartesian refusal to give up on duality. Duality rejects the monist perspective that the brain constitutes the mind, instead valorizing the concept that the mind is something distinctive and beyond the body (Bunge, 1991). Descartes proposed that the human experience was defined by having a mind which he called "the soul," distinct from but related to the body. Descartes's notion of dualism as a philosophical position is compatible with most theologies, which claim that the soul exists, that it is immortal, and that there exists an afterlife distinct from life within the physical world (Hart, 1996). The mind and the body are viewed as separate entities with different life courses and duration.

In recent years, research has validated that the mind-body connection is relevant to psychology, as processes of the brain have been shown to have striking manifestations in the body. Some of the most compelling research has involved complex trauma. Complex trauma during childhood is a prevalent and important predictor of both child and adult psychopathology, as well as a number of somatic disorders (Anda et al., 2006; Kessler et al., 2010; Shonkoff, 2011). Survivors of childhood complex trauma have been found to have a higher incidence of abnormalities of white matter integrity in the corpus callosum (CC) (Rinne-Albers et al., 2016). The CC is the neural structure that connects the left and right hemispheres of the brain, providing the central pathway for facilitating the flow of information from one side of the brain to the other (Shapiro & Forrest, 2016). De Bellis et al. (1999) have argued that impairments to the CC resulting from complex trauma represent a pre-existing vulnerability and are predictive of pathologic vulnerability to psychological trauma and the eventual development of PTSD (Gilbertson et al., 2002). A substantial body of empirical work evidences the psychophysiological and somatic comorbidities of PTSD (Shapiro & Forrest, 2016; Rinne-Albers et al., 2016; Anda et al., 2006; Kessler et al., 2010).

All of these findings challenge the notion of Cartesian dualism, as we shift toward viewing PTSD as a systematic disorder rather than just a disorder of the mind (McFarlane, 2017). This systematic view of the mind and the body relates more to monism rather that the concept of dualism. The monist perspective of the mind-body relationship proposed that there is only one unifying reality: The mind and the body are to be treated and understood as one entity, a whole. Assuming that the brain and the mind are one, complex trauma treatment should also be holistic, integrative, and inclusive of both the mind and the body. Treatment of complex trauma has evolved into a more integrative, body-oriented approach through modalities such as Eye Movement Desensitization and Reprocessing (Shapiro, 1989), Sensorimotor Psychotherapy (Ogden & Minton, 2000), and Somatic Experiencing (Levine, 1997), each offering interventions that can be used autonomously by clients to enhance self-empowered healing of the body and the mind (described in-depth in Chap. 8).

The Modulation Model

A central feature of complex trauma is a loss of the ability to physiologically modulate stress as well as diminished capacity to utilize bodily signals (van der Kolk et al., 1996). The threat of trauma triggers a cascade of both psychological and physical defenses, which are designed to evaluate and reduce stress and maximize the chances for survival (van der Hart & Nijenhuis, 1999). A foundational part of complex trauma treatment is to begin to enhance the trauma survivor's awareness of affective states which relate to emotion, motivational intensity (the urge to move toward/away from a stimulus), and the level of arousal measured subjectively (Bradley & Lang, 2007; O'Shea Brown, 2021). For instance, if you were unlucky enough to be *chased* by a bear, your "flight" response would kick in, and you would run as fast as possible. If asked to rate your level of fear in that moment, you would probably put it close to a 10 out of 10. Your heart would race and your palms would sweat, signs that your sympathetic nervous system is fully activated. Upon reaching safety, your body would take some time to return to normal functioning. Survivors of complex trauma, however, may have the same physiological response not to a bear or other obvious physical threat, but to an abusive parent or partner who triggers a similar level of arousal because of a history of physical or emotional abuse that has taken place repeatedly for a prolonged period.

In cases of prolonged relational trauma, living in a constant fight/flight response state is not adaptive over time. Consequently, survivors of complex trauma often present with increased dissociative symptoms and may feel disconnected or numb and alienated from their body and emotions (as discussed in Chap. 5). Establishing safety in the body is paramount to the healing process for complex trauma. The Modulation Model (Ogden et al., 2006) offers a multipurpose conceptual framework to assess present experience of regulation/dysregulation and the accompanying intense emotions. For instance, the emotions of stress and/or fear are necessary for survival, as they enable us to assess for threat, and determine resources for intervention and safety. However, intense negative emotions can linger in the mind and the body long after the threat of the trauma has passed. The Modulation Model offers a measure of regulation and dysregulation, enabling the clinician and the client to assess the level of arousal and affective state together (as shown in Fig. 6.1).

Within the Modulation Model, there are three arousal states: hyperarousal, hypoarousal, and the optimal arousal zone referred to as the "window of tolerance," a term coined by Siegel (1999) (Table 6.1). Together these states describe the body's responses to stress. Arousal refers to physiological functioning that determines our level of awareness (how alert one is to their environment). Trauma occurs when an individual is overwhelmed by something that is out of their control. When an individual leaves their optimal arousal state or window of tolerance, the body experiences dysregulation in the form of hypoarousal or hyperarousal. Hyperarousal, otherwise known as the fight/flight response, is evident in such indicators as heart rate, breath rate, muscle tension, and impulse for movement (Ogden & Minton, 2000; Siegel, 1999). Hypoarousal may occur when we have too much hyperarousal, surpassing the pain that our body is able to tolerate, causing us to plunge into a state of shutting down or dissociating. The survival instinct is either to become hyperalert and aware or to become numb, very similar to primal surrender in the animal kingdom (Ogden & Minton, 2000). Primal surrender, also known colloquially as "playing dead," is a behavior in which animals take on the appearance of being dead as a defense mechanism to adaptively allow them to escape a situation where the supposed predator is too large to fight or too quick to flee from.

By utilizing this model in the psychoeducation component of your treatment plan, you provide a client with a heightened sense of awareness of the body's responses to stress. They can then begin to focus on building affect tolerance through mindfulness, that is, the ability to notice a feeling state or bodily sensation and accompanying emotions. When an individual leaves their optimal arousal state or

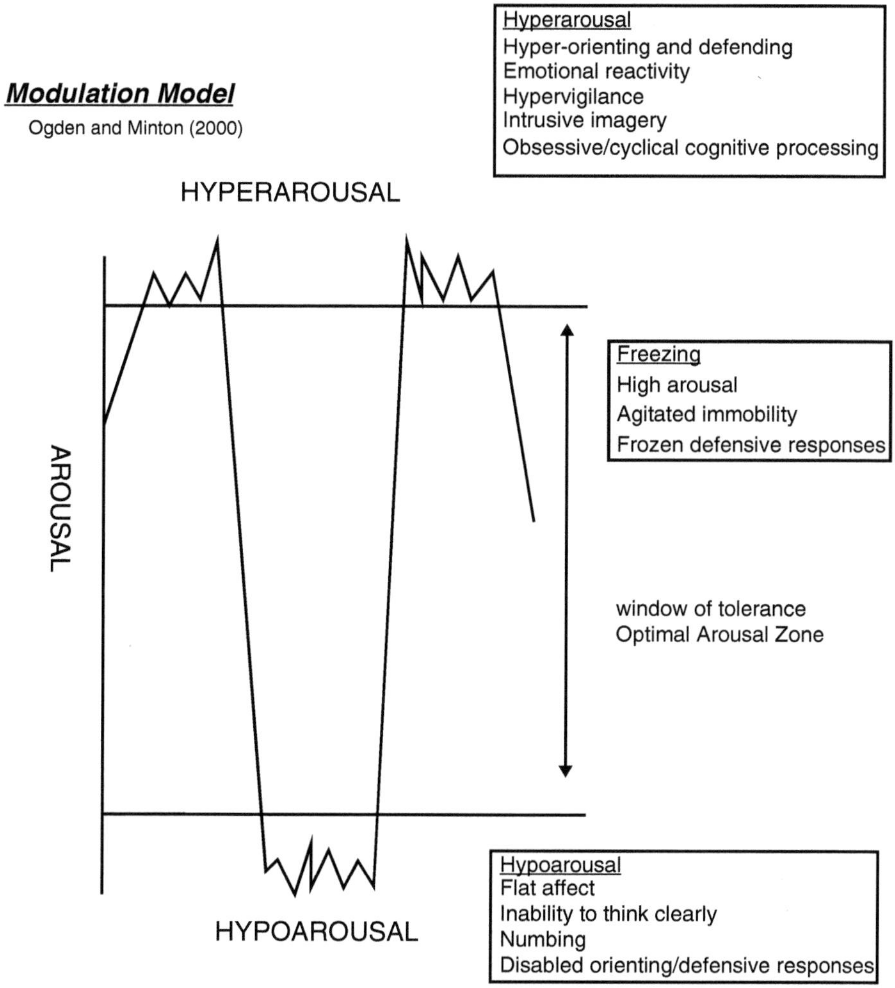

Fig. 6.1 The Modulation Model. [Copyright © 2000 by American Psychological Association. Reproduced with permission. Ogden, P., & Minton, K. (2000). Sensorimotor psychotherapy: One method for processing traumatic memory. *Traumatology*, 6(3), 149–173. https://doi.org/10.1177/153476560000600302]

window of tolerance, the body experiences dysregulation in the form of hypoarousal or hyperarousal. If you cannot manage the emotions of stress or its physical symptoms, you will begin to experience fight, flight, or freeze responses. Being aware of the window of tolerance allows an individual to better manage mental health and gauge their sense of safety around particular situations or people. For example, when a client experiences hyperarousal in the presence of an abrasive or emotionally abusive colleague, they may experience symptoms of shortness of breath, racing thoughts, and a sense of panic. In this instance, their body is not betraying them,

Table 6.1 Signs and symptoms of dissociation in a clinical setting

Arousal states	Signs and symptoms may include:
Hyperarousal	Impulses to frantically reach for help, flee, or fight
	Intense emotions, e.g., anger, irritability, and fear
	Sleep disturbance
	Difficulty concentrating
	Constantly feeling on-guard (hypervigilance)
	Heightened impulsivity
	Muscle tension
	Increased heart rate
	Feeling "jumpy" (startle response is easily activated)
	Shortness of breath
	Flashbacks/intrusive thoughts or images
	Unable to process stimuli effectively
Hypoarousal	Disconnected from emotions
	Memory fragmentation
	Numbing
	Dissociation (distance from self, body, or emotions)
	Sleep disturbance
	Difficulty concentrating
	Low energy
	Flat affect
	Unable to process stimuli effectively
Optimal arousal (the window of tolerance)	Feeling present in the moment
	Ability to adaptively self-soothe (mindfulness, breath work)
	Emotionally regulated/ability to regulate emotions
	Feeling safe
	Feeling in control
	Slow rhythmic breathing
	Cognitive flexibility

but rather adaptively alerting and preparing them to leave a toxic situation, similar to the bear analogy mentioned earlier. Some individuals misinterpret these signals of self-protection and begin to maladaptively self-soothe as a means to "switch off" hyperarousal.

Ritualized compulsive comfort-seeking, what traditionalists call addiction, is a relatively common response to the adversity experienced in childhood, emerging as a coping behavior for survivors who were never taught healthy alternatives to managing stress when they were young (Derefinko et al., 2019). Adversity in childhood is highly correlated to addiction in adulthood as many survivors of complex trauma feel dysregulated much of the time (Shonkoff et al., 2012; Substance Abuse and Mental Health Services Administration, 2018). However, this maladaptive behavioral pattern can cause further pain, shame, and re-traumatization. Recognizing dysregulation will provide you and your client with the opportunity to understand triggers, symptoms, and emotional needs. When fight, flight, or freeze responses are activated, adaptive strategies such as the integration of somatic-based therapies, breath work, and mindfulness can be applied to re-enter the window of tolerance (Fisher, 2002; van der Kolk, 1996a). Over time this promotes the ability to widen the window of tolerance, which, in turn, will increase the client's sense of calm and their agency to deal with stress through the more adaptive approach of becoming regulated.

Polyvagal Theory

Polyvagal Theory offers a conceptual framework for understanding the relationship between autonomic subsystems and the regulation of social behaviors, by providing a method of understanding and appreciating that our nervous system responds to challenges adaptively. Therefore, teaching this theory to trauma survivors in a clinical setting will assist them in depathologizing physiological symptoms of trauma and promote positive regard toward the body. The theory also provides clinicians with a useful picture of the three-part nervous system which includes the response systems we are already familiar with: immobilization (i.e., playing dead, promoted by the dorsal vagus nerve) and mobilization (i.e., fight-or-flight response behaviors, promoted by the sympathetic nervous system). The theory also identifies a third type of nervous system response that Porges (2003) calls the "social engagement system." The social engagement system describes a playful combination of activation and calming that operates out of a unique nerve influence, the ventral vagal. The ventral vagal is responsible for displaying facial expressions, mirroring, attunement, empathy, and eye contact (Porges, 2009). The three-part nervous system described in Polyvagal Theory can be viewed in Fig. 6.2.

When trauma occurs, the dorsal vagal system suppresses the sympathetic and social engagement system; similarly, the sympathetic system inhibits the social engagement system, and the social engagement system has the capacity to down-regulate the sympathetic system (Porges, 2003). This means the dorsal vagal system is designed as a protective reflex, an attempt to defend the self from possible physical and psychic harm in a bid to ensure survival. This framework connects neurophysiological patterns of autonomic regulation with expression of emotional and social behavior. It provides a helpful means of understanding the human response to trauma and how this manifests through behavior, stress, and illness. When a client is chronically activated (sympathetic state), it can be challenging to assist them in regulating their body back into the "window of tolerance" or ventral vagal.

It is important for the clinician to be mindful of the significance of their own affective state, which can serve as an anchor for the client, helping them to feel settled (O'Shea Brown, 2021). The calm, nurturing presence of the clinician serves as a support in guiding the client to co-regulate and observe their stress responses in a curious and compassionate way. When a client is encouraged to notice the sensations of their protective responses, they are less focused on fighting or suppressing

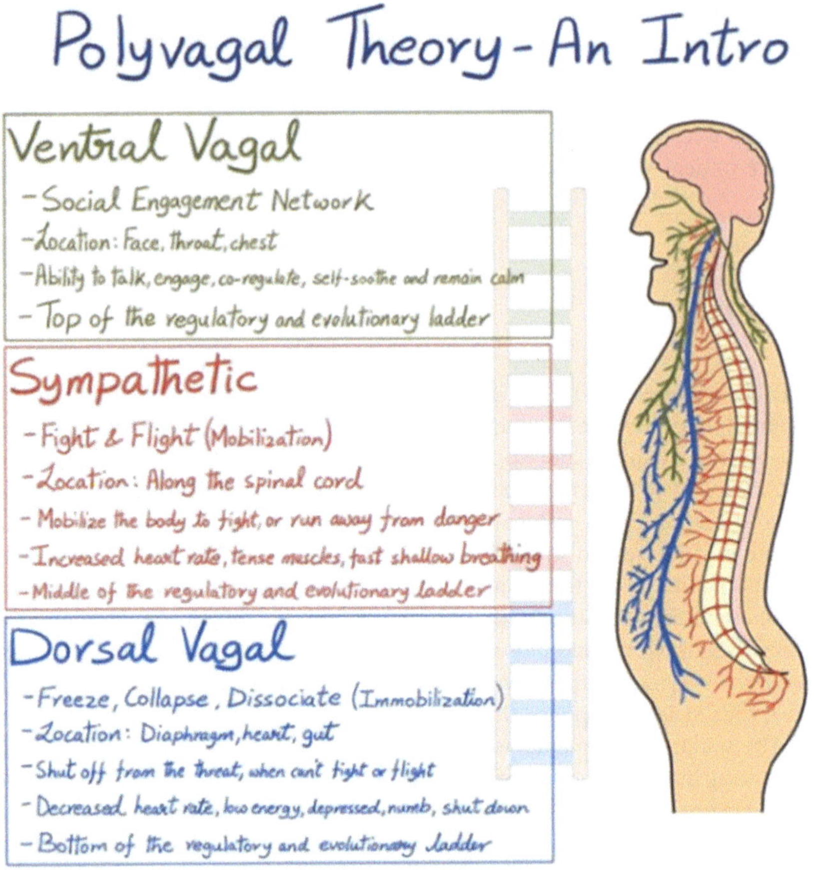

Fig. 6.2 Polyvagal Theory (Credit: Illustration sourced by EMDR-trained Psychotherapist © Ayan Mukherjee – therapyillustrated.com, used with permission). Ayan Mukherjee is a registered psychotherapist and EMDRIA-approved certified EMDR therapist and Consultant-in-Training, with a private practice in Toronto, Canada. Mukherjee is the creator of the illustrations on Polyvagal Theory and EMDR Reprocessing Phase that have been used in this book. For more information about visual aid tools for trauma therapy: www.TherapyIllustrated.com

them and more interested in understanding and appreciating how this primitive protective response system attempts to serve them. In short, the body becomes their friend rather than their foe, their protector rather than their unpredictable, irrational enemy, and their knowledge of the mind-body connection can begin to evolve.

Somatization and Implicit Memory

Implicit memory describes the process by which past experiences are remembered without conscious effort. One of its common forms is procedural memory. For instance, we access our procedural memory when brushing our teeth, bicycling, and even driving. Actions that rely on implicit memory are supported by previous experiences, classic conditioning, and priming. Regardless of how long ago experiences occurred, individuals can perform the tasks stored as implicit memory without conscious effort. For example, if individuals learn how to balance on a bicycle in childhood, this information is automatically available to us in adulthood. Similarly, survivors of relational trauma hold an implicit memory of traumatic events in both the mind and body (Rothschild, 2000), such that the body may remember a traumatic event even if the individual cannot consciously recall the details (Rothschild, 2000; Schore, 2002; van der Kolk, 1994). In other words, early relational trauma is experienced through emotional and physiological responses which are encoded into implicit memory.

Individuals who have experienced early relational trauma may associate emotional need and vulnerability with suffering. For example, a child may remember the pain and distress of being ignored and rejected by an unavailable, dismissive parent. In these circumstances, reaching out for love or support may become paired with rejection and inadequacy. The internal experience can manifest through a negative self-belief, such as "My needs are not being met because I am unlovable." Rothschild (2000) suggests that every sensory modality is encoded as somatic information in traumatic memory. These somatic experiences can be triggered when similar conditions are present, even if the origin cannot be recalled. This means that as that child grows older, they may carry the negative self-concept that vulnerability leads to rejection and may therefore operate from a place of classic conditioning rather than deeper self-awareness. The ignored child may see the world as a dreadful place – they may become distrusting and defensive in close relationships as the conditioned negative beliefs become self-fulfilling prophecies. A traumatized person's perception of reality may become distorted such that they feel imprisoned in a perpetual reliving of their deepest pain, again, even if the individual does not consciously recall or express the past events (O'Shea Brown, 2020). Traumatic memories in early childhood can be stored in the amygdala in implicit form, and these affective states remain dissociated from the trauma survivor's consciousness while continuing to influence behavior and thought in powerful ways (Simpkins & Simpkins, 2010).

A traumatized individual's memory can be expressed through persistent fear, constriction of movement, and a range of somatic symptoms (Johnson, 2009; Levine, 1997). Somatization is defined as psychological distress in the form of physical symptoms, including chest pain, fatigue, dizziness, headache, edema, back pain, shortness of breath, abdominal pain, or numbness (Kroenke & Mangelsdorff, 1989). Research by Barkley and colleagues (2005) found that approximately 20% of patients who present to primary care doctors experience physical symptoms that have a purely psychological cause (i.e., psychosomatic symptoms). One of the main goals of trauma-informed therapy is to facilitate individuals to better understand their bodily sensations by verbally identifying and describing these sensations in a meaningful narrative (Rothschild, 2000). For instance, the client who experiences a tightness in the throat during public speaking may associate this physical sensation with the core negative concept, "I am stupid." When asked to name an earlier memory involving this sensation, they recall the previous experience of floundering over words at a spelling bee. Even though this memory is not readily available in the conscious mind, the implicit memory provides a somatic cue anytime that person is at risk of feeling inadequate or imprudent.

Autoimmune Disorders

The Adverse Childhood Experiences Study (ACES) sought to understand how adversity in the formative years goes on to impede healthy development and wellness in adulthood (Felitti et al., 1998). This study found that adult survivors of clustered adverse childhood experiences were at increased risk of developing chronic health problems, mental illness, and substance misuse in adulthood. The study found that most people (approximately 64%) score positive on at least one item on the ACE scale and 12% of the population have an ACE score of 4 or more, which doubles the risk of heart disease and cancer. It increases the likelihood of becoming an alcoholic by 700% and the risk of attempted suicide by 1200% (CDC, 2014; Felitti et al., 1998). The somatic pathologies associated with adverse experiences in the formative years range from poor physical health to higher instances of autoimmune disorders and addictive behaviors. Therefore, trauma not only impacts mental health but also deeply impacts physiological well-being and overall health. Increasing evidence suggests a link between posttraumatic stress disorder (PTSD) and physical health stress disorders, which may lead to impairment of the immune system and subsequent autoimmune disease (Bookwalter et al., 2020). Bookwalter et al. (2020) found that PTSD is highly correlated with heightened risk of autoimmune diseases such as rheumatoid arthritis, systemic lupus, erythematosus, inflammatory bowel diseases, and multiple sclerosis.

When a person is experiencing pervasive hypervigilance and stress regarding ongoing or retrospective abuse, neglect, fear, or deprivation, bodily systems break down. In the short term, inflammation serves as a physiological mechanism of self-protection. However, it is a serious threat if activated chronically. Chronic inflammation can lead to a variety of illnesses, including diabetes, cardiovascular disease, arthritis, cancer, dementia, and depression (Danese & McEwen, 2012). Since inflammation has been linked to multiple diseases, the fact that early life adversity is associated with elevated inflammatory responses suggests that toxic stress increases the probability of lifelong health impairment (Danese & McEwen, 2012). Trauma, PTSD, and chronic stress generate an alertness to threat and a feeling of lack of safety in which mental processing falls second to adaptive survival responses (Williamson et al., 2015). It has been hypothesized that an association between PTSD and autoimmune disease may be at least partially explained by unhealthy behaviors such as the aforementioned ritualistic compulsive comfort-seeking in substance abuse. However, this does not take away from the burden of pain, fear, and shame that is carried by the survivor in their body and in their mind.

Summary

It has been established that exposure to the threat of trauma stimulates the autonomic nervous system, resulting in sympathetic hyperarousal and parasympathetic hypoarousal states that accompany the survival responses of fight, flight, submission, and freeze (LeDoux, 2002; Ogden et al., 2006; Porges, 2003; van der Kolk, 1996a, 1996b). For this reason, the treatment of complex trauma should be phase-oriented, multimodal, and skill-focused, with a core emphasis on symptom relief and functional improvement. Understanding the body through the lens of the Modulation Model and Polyvagal Theory can equip the clinician to provide psychoeducation to their clients, with a view to depathologizing physiological responses to trauma. This allows the survivor to operate out of deep self-awareness rather than classic conditioning. It is critical for therapists to build strong attunement and observation skills to attune to a client's level of arousal. From here the therapeutic focus can gravitate toward grounding techniques to empower the client to manage their symptoms outside of the therapy room.

Questions and Activities for Discussion and Further Reflection

1. What are the core differences between hyperarousal and hypoarousal?
2. Do you understand the window of tolerance?
3. Can you provide a brief synopsis of Polyvagal Theory?
4. Can you describe the following terms: (i) somatization and (ii) implicit memory?

Exercise

1. *Class is invited to engage in a grounding exercise as directed by professor. Afterward there will be a discussion on any sensations or changes in affective state before and after.*

References

Anda, R. F., Felitti, V. J., Bremner, J. D., Walker, J. D., Whitfield, C., Perry, B. D., … Giles, W. H. (2006). The enduring effects of abuse and related adverse experiences in childhood. A convergence of evidence from neurobiology and epidemiology. *European Archives of Psychiatry and Clinical Neuroscience, 256*, 174–186. https://doi.org/10.1007/s00406-005-0624-4

Bookwalter, D., Roenfeldt, K, LeardMann, C. et al. Posttraumatic stress disorder and risk of selected autoimmune diseases among US military personnel. BMC Psychiatry 20, 23 (2020). https://doi.org/10.1186/s12888-020-2432-9

Bradley, M. M., & Lang, P. J. (2007). Emotion and motivation. In J. T. Cacioppo, L. G. Tassinary, & G. Berntson (Eds.), *Handbook of psychophysiology* (Vol. 5, 3rd ed., pp. 81–607). New York, NY: Cambridge University Press.

Briere, J., & Scott, C. (2006). *Principles of trauma therapy: A guide to symptoms, evaluation, and treatment*. London, UK: Sage.

Bunge, M. (1991). A philosophical perspective on the mind-body problem or, why neuroscientists and psychologists should care about philosophy. *Proceedings of the American Philosophical Society, 135*(4), 513–523.

Centers for Disease Control and Prevention, National Center for Injury Prevention and Control, Division of Violence Prevention. (2014, May). *The Adverse Childhood Experiences (ACE) Study*. cdc.gov. Atlanta, Georgia. Archived from the original on 27 December 2015.

Chessick, R. D. (2009). Implications of the current insolubility of the mind-brain problem for the contemporary practice of psychodynamic psychiatry. *Journal of the American Academy of Psychoanalysis and Dynamic Psychiatry, 37*(2), 315–352.

Courtois, C. A., Ford, J. D., & Cloitre, M. (2009). Best practices in psychotherapy for adults. In C. A. Courtois & J. D. Ford (Eds.), *Treating complex traumatic stress disorders; an evidence-based guide* (pp. 82–103). New York, NY: Guilford Press.

Crane, T. (1999). Mind-body problem. In R. A. Wilson & F. Keil (Eds.), *The MIT Encyclopedia of the cognitive sciences* (pp. 546–548). Cambridge, MA: MIT Press.

Danese, A., & McEwen, B. S. (2012). Adverse childhood experiences, allostasis, allostatic load, and age-related disease. *Physiology and Behavior, 106*(1), 29–39.

De Bellis, M. D., Keshavan, M., Clark, D. B., Casey, B. J., Giedd, J., Boring, A. M., … Bennett, A. E. (1999). Research award. Developmental traumatology, part II: Brain development. *Biological Psychiatry, 45*, 1271–1284.

Derefinko, K. J., Salgado García, F. I., Talley, K. M., Bursac, Z., Johnson, K. C., Murphy, J. G., … Sumrok, D. D. (2019). Adverse childhood experiences predict opioid relapse during treatment among rural adults. *Addictive Behaviors, 96*, 171–174. https://doi.org/10.1016/j.addbeh.2019.05.008

Felitti, V. J., Anda, R. F., Nordenberg, D., Williamson, D. F., Spitz, A. M., Edwards, V., … Marks, J. S. (1998). Relationship of childhood abuse and household dysfunction to many of the leading causes of death in adults. The adverse childhood experiences (ACE) study. *American Journal of Preventive Medicine, 14*, 245–258.

Fisher, J. (2002). *Adapting EMDR Techniques in the treatment of dysregulated or dissociative patients*. Paper presented at the International Society for the Study of Dissociation Annual Meeting, San Antonio, Texas November 12, 2000.

Gerdes, K. E., Segal, E. A., & Harmon, J. K. (2013). Your brain on empathy: Implications for social work practice. In H. C. Matto & M. Ballan (Eds.), *Neuroscience for social work: Current research and practice*. New York, NY: Springer Publishing Company.

Gilbertson, M. W., Shenton, M. E., Ciszewski, A., Kasai, K., Lasko, N. B., Orr, S. P., & Pitman, R. K. (2002). Smaller hippocampal volume predicts pathologic vulnerability to psychological trauma. *Nature Neuroscience, 5*(11), 1242–1247. https://doi.org/10.1038/nn958

Hart, W. D. (1996). Dualism. In S. Guttenplan (Ed.), *A companion to the philosophy of mind* (pp. 265–267). Oxford, UK: Blackwell.

Johnson, R. (2009). Oppression embodied: The intersecting dimensions of trauma, oppression, and somatic psychology. The U.S.A. *Body Psychotherapy Journal, 8*(1), 19–31.

Kessler, R. C., McLaughlin, K. A., Green, J. G., Gruber, M. J., Sampson, N. A., Zaslavsky, A. M., … Williams, D. R. (2010). Childhood adversities and adult psychopathology in the WHO world mental health surveys. *The British Journal of Psychiatry, 197*, 378–385. https://doi.org/10.1192/bjp.bp.110.080499

Kroenke, K., & Mangelsdorff, A. D. (1989). Common symptoms in ambulatory care: Incidence, evaluation, therapy, and outcome. *The American Journal of Medicine, 86*(3), 262–266. https://doi.org/10.1016/0002-9343(89)90293-3

LeDoux, J. (2002). *The synaptic self: How our brains become who we are*. New York, NY: Guilford Press.

Levine, P. (1997). *Waking the Tiger: Healing trauma*. Berkeley, CA: North Atlantic Books.

Lowenstein, R., & Goodwin, J. (1999). Assessment and management of somatoform symptoms in traumatized patients: Conceptual overview and pragmatic guide. In J. Goodwin & R. Attias (Eds.), *Splintered reflection: Images of the body in trauma* (pp. 67–88). New York, NY: Basic Books.

McFarlane, A. C. (2017). Post-traumatic stress disorder is a systemic illness, not a mental disorder: Is Cartesian dualism dead? *The Medical Journal of Australia, 206*(6), 248–249. https://doi.org/10.5694/mja17.00048

O'Shea Brown, G. (2020). Internal family systems informed eye movement desensitization and reprocessing: An integrative technique for treatment of complex posttraumatic stress disorder. *International Body Psychotherapy Journal, 19*(2), 112–122.

O'Shea Brown, G. (2021). Reflections on providing virtual eye movement desensitization and reprocessing therapy in the wake of COVID-19: Survival through adaptation. In C. Tosone (Ed.), *Shared trauma, shared resilience during a pandemic: Social work in the time of COVID-19*. Cham, Switzerland: Springer.

Ogden, P., & Minton, K. (2000). Sensorimotor psychotherapy: One method for processing traumatic memory. *Traumatology, VI*(3), article 3.

Ogden, P., Minton, K., & Pain, C. (2006). *Trauma and the body: A sensorimotor approach to psychotherapy*. New York, NY: Norton.

Porges, S. W. (2003). The polyvagal theory: Phylogenetic contributions to social behavior. *Physiology & Behavior, 79*, 503–513.

Porges, S. W. (2009). The polyvagal theory: New insights into adaptive reactions of the autonomic nervous system. *Cleveland Clinic Journal of Medicine, 76*(Suppl 2), S86–S90. Available at: http://www-ncbi-nlm-nih-gov.proxy.library.nyu.edu/pubmed/19376991

Rinne-Albers, M. A., van der Werff, S. J., van Hoof, M. J., van Lang, N. D., Lamers-Winkelman, F., Rombouts, S. A., … van der Wee, N. J. (2016). Abnormalities of white matter integrity in the corpus callosum of adolescents with PTSD after childhood sexual abuse: A DTI study. *European Child & Adolescent Psychiatry, 25*(8), 869–878. https://doi.org/10.1007/s00787-015-0805-2

Rothschild, B. (2000). *The body remembers. The psychophysiology of trauma and trauma treatment*. New York, NY: W. W. Norton.

Schore, A. (2002). Dysregulation of the right brain: A fundamental mechanism of traumatic attachment and the psychopathogenesis of posttraumatic stress disorder. *Australian and New Zealand Journal of Psychiatry, 36*, 9–30.

Searle, J. R. (2002). Why I am not a property dualist. *Journal of Consciousness Studies, 9*(12), 57–64.

Shapiro, F. (1989). Efficacy of the eye movement desensitization procedure in the treatment of traumatic memories. *Journal of Traumatic Stress., 2*(2), 199–223. https://doi.org/10.1002/jts.2490020207

Shapiro, F., & Forrest, M. S. (2016). *EMDR: Breakthrough therapy for overcoming anxiety, stress & trauma*. New York, NY: Basic Books.

Shonkoff, J. P. (2011). Protecting brains, not simply stimulating minds. *Science, 333*, 982–983. https://doi.org/10.1126/science.1206014

Shonkoff, J. P., Garner, A. S., Siegel, B. S., Dobbins, M. I., Earls, M. F., McGuinn, L., & Care, D. (2012). The lifelong effects of early childhood adversity and toxic stress. *Pediatrics, 129*(1), e232–e246.

Siegel, D. J. (1999). *The developing mind: toward a neurobiology of interpersonal experience*. New York: Guilford Press.

Simpkins, A., & Simpkins, A. M. (2010). *The Dao of neuroscience: Combining eastern and western principles for optimal therapeutic change*. New York, NY: WW Norton and Company.

Substance Abuse and Mental Health Services Administration. (2018). *The role of adverse childhood experiences in substance abuse and related behavioral health problems*. Retrieved from https://www-samhsa-gov.proxy.library.nyu.edu/capt/sites/default/files/resources/aces-behavioral-health-problems.pdf. Accessed 5 March 19.

van der Kolk, B. A. (1994). The body keeps the score: Memory and the evolving psychobiology of posttraumatic stress. *Harvard Review of Psychiatry, 1*(5), 253–265.

van der Kolk, B. A. (1996a). *The complexity of adaptation to trauma: Self-regulation, stimulus discrimination, and characterological development. Traumatic stress: The effects of overwhelming experience on mind, body, and society* (pp. 182–213). New York, NY: Guilford Press.

van der Kolk, B. A. (1996b). The body keeps the score: Approaches to the psychobiology of posttraumatic stress disorder. In *Traumatic stress: The effects of overwhelming experience on mind, body, and society* (pp. 214–241). New York, NY: Guilford Press.

van der Kolk, B. A., McFarlane, A., & Weisaeth, L. (1996). *Traumatic stress*. New York, NY: Guilford.

van der Hart, O., & Nijenhuis, E. R. S. (1999). Bearing witness to uncorroborated trauma: The clinician's development of reflective belief. *Professional Psychology: Research and Practice, 30*(1), 37–44.

Williamson, J. B., Porges, E. C., Lamb, D. G., & Porges, S. W. (2015). Maladaptive autonomic regulation in PTSD accelerates physiological aging. *Frontiers in psychology, 5*, 1571. https://doi.org/10.3389/fpsyg.2014.01571

Chapter 7
The Power of Belief

A sense of self begins in the formative years, influenced from birth through infancy by attachment figures and other role models. Eventually identity and personality become more solidified in adulthood, as do our beliefs (Bowlby, 1980; Kirshner, 1991; Kohut, 1977; Richards, 1982). Our beliefs shape our lives and relationships in many powerful ways. They represent what we hold to be true and are often supported by statements, observations, and events that we have experienced in our environments. Beliefs can be categorized into spheres, such as political, religious, societal, ideological, and, most importantly, core self-beliefs. Our belief system informs our perception of reality, our choices, and our experiences of the world, which cumulatively inform our perception of ourselves. We have all heard of "the power of belief" or intrinsically felt that power within us in some form or another. The power of belief is most evident in occurrences of placebo and radical remission. Moseley et al. (2002) investigated this phenomenon by conducting a randomized, placebo-controlled trial to evaluate the efficacy of arthroscopy for osteoarthritis of the knee. Many patients report symptomatic relief after undergoing arthroscopy of the knee for osteoarthritis, but experts were unclear how the procedure achieves this result. Moseley et al. were curious about the role of belief in the healing process.

A sample group of 180 patients presenting with a diagnosis of osteoarthritis of the knee were recruited to participate in the study. Participants were randomly divided into three groups: one group received arthroscopic debridement, another group received arthroscopic lavage, and the third group had placebo surgery. Patients in the placebo group received skin incisions and underwent a simulated debridement without insertion of the arthroscope. Patients and assessors of outcome were blinded to the treatment received. Outcomes were assessed at multiple points over a 24-month period with the use of five self-reported scores and one objective test of walking and stair climbing. A total of 165 patients completed the trial. Astonishingly, at no point did either of the intervention groups report less pain or better function than the placebo group, even 1 year later. The conclusion of this study was that the brain believed the body would heal and so it did. Experiences create thoughts and

G. O'Shea Brown, *Healing Complex Posttraumatic Stress Disorder*, Essential Clinical Social Work Series, https://doi.org/10.1007/978-3-030-61416-4_7

thoughts become metabolized into memory, perception, and identity. Beliefs become stronger and even more deeply rooted when they are repeatedly affirmed by our environment or attachment figures.

In this study, the patients believed they were being cared for, believed they were being monitored, and expected to get better. Conversely, when our environment and experiences suggest we will not be cared for, this creates negative expectations that also color our reality. This chapter will begin by reviewing how core negative beliefs form in the unconscious mind before reviewing the role bias plays in shaping an individual's reality. Subsequently this chapter will explore how beliefs contribute to the psychological phenomenon in which individuals display inclination to re-enact traumatic or painful events; how beliefs impact experiences in close relationships will also be considered. Finally, this chapter will review how blocking beliefs can be linked to memories from which they are formed, in addition to exploring how self-determination impacts the clinical process.

Core Negative Self-Beliefs

Bowlby (1989) hypothesized that a child's earliest experiences with their parents lead to the development of core beliefs regarding self-worth, safety, security, and the trustworthiness of others, which he termed *the internal working model.* Children make sense of the world by creating emotional maps to assist them in discerning who they should trust and how they will survive. When children's needs are adequately met, they can begin to develop trust that the world is an intrinsically benevolent place (Bowlby, 1980). However, in the event of pervasive relational trauma in childhood, such as rejection, humiliation, or neglect, children can develop beliefs which negatively affect their ability to establish a sense of safety and maintain healthy relationships (Lee & Hankin, 2009; Main & Hesse, 1990; van IJzendoorn, 1995). Trauma informs identity, not just through the development of maladaptive behaviors such as hypervigilance and psychological reactivity or numbing to sensitivity cues but also through the formation of shame-based cognition also known as core negative beliefs (Shapiro & Forrest, 2016).

As we navigate our early relationships and environments, we begin to make meaning of our experiences, and from here core beliefs are formed. Many children will adopt a moral defense as a coping strategy, blaming themselves for their parent's ineffective parenting. Fairbairn (1943) originated "the Moral Defense Against Bad Objects," explaining that it was a defensive strategy applied by children to lessen their anxiety about being dependent on objects who continuously frustrated their needs. This strategy preserves the biologically needed attachment to the parent. The children Dr. Fairbairn studied were obviously neglected and came from abusive families; however, they vehemently defended their parents when he questioned them about the abuse. He was astonished by how eager the abused children were to blame themselves for the neglect and/or abuse. They internalized the "badness" of their parental objects as a defensive strategy. Children have such limited

Table 7.1 Examples of core positive beliefs and negative beliefs

Negative self-beliefs	Positive self-beliefs
I am not worthy of love	*I deserve love*
I am unlovable	*I am lovable*
I am a bad person	*I am a good person*
I am not good enough	*I am good enough (just as I am)*
I am ugly	*I am desirable/attractive*
I am stupid	*I am capable*
I do not matter	*I matter in the world (it's okay to ask for what I need)*
I deserve to be miserable	*I deserve to be happy*
I am insignificant	*I am worthy and worthwhile*
It is all my fault	*What happened does not define me/it was not my fault*
I cannot be trusted	*I am trustworthy*
I am a freak	*I am special and unique*
I am not safe	*I am safe now/the risk of harm has passed*
I am incompetent	*I am capable/competent*
I am irresponsible	*I have evolved into a responsible adult/I am learning to be accountable and consistent*
I have to be perfect/I have to please everyone	*I can ask for what I need and still be liked/lovable*
I am not in control	*I am now in control*
I am a failure (and always will be)	*I can achieve and succeed*

control and agency in their lives that they adopt the moral defense in an attempt to assume a heightened sense of control and responsibility, even for traumatic events. Although traumatic events in the formative years are incidents that the child simply has no control over, the child will internalize his, her, or their central negative belief. This is what leads to the development of shame-based cognition.

All individuals have global meanings: broad schemas of what they expect in the world, in their relationships, and of themselves, shaped by their history and influenced by their core beliefs (O'Shea Brown, 2020). A child who has endured numerous experiences of rejection by the attachment figure has a memory network which indicates to them that they are in some way not good enough. The experience of trauma in the formative years generates painful memories which inform core negative self-beliefs. Therefore, clients presenting with C-PTSD will have complex relationships with themselves and others. Core beliefs can be both positive and negative. For examples, see Table 7.1.

Negativity Bias and Confirmation Bias

Our belief system informs our perception of reality, our choices, and our experiences of the world. Beliefs become stronger and even more deeply rooted when they are repeatedly affirmed by our environment. A bias is a tendency or inclination toward a particular belief system; some biases can be positive and helpful, and others may cause harm (Munroe et al., 1997). Negativity bias is the principle that "negative events are more salient, potent, dominant in combinations, and generally efficacious than positive events" (Rozin & Royzman, 2001, p. 297). We are all evolutionarily wired to have a negativity bias, which was adaptive in early human societies: Our ancestors who were hunter-gatherers were safer by assuming that there was a lion around every corner. The ones lurking in the tall grass looking for the predatory lion survived, while those sunning themselves on the warm rock were devoured. Thus, a certain proclivity to think negatively is handed down from our ancestors. This manifests in ways big and small.

For example, if you took a young child to the zoo, bought them an ice cream, and watched the polar bears, it would be a fun and enjoyable day. However, if on the way home the child is stung by a bee on the tongue while eating the ice cream, this day will likely be preserved in the child's memory as the day they were stung by a bee on the tongue. Ice cream may even become associated with physical pain and the feeling state of powerlessness. We have a much stronger propensity to absorb and preserve memory and associations comprised of negative stimuli than those comprised of positive stimuli. The more intense the negative elements of the memory, and the more attention we paid to them at the time, the more dominant those elements in our recollection. Cacioppo, Cacioppo, and Gollan (2014) explain that negative stimuli create a strong surge of neurological activity in the amygdala, an area of the brain designed for critical processing. This is a reflexive and protective way to ensure safety; however, it also means that painful memories take precedence over positive associations (Cacioppo et al., 2014; Rozin & Royzman, 2001).

Though it is possible to change our beliefs, it is very challenging. This reticence to discard old beliefs can be attributed to confirmation bias, a principle which posits that humans have an unconscious propensity to search for, favor, recall, and interpret information in a way that confirms their previous beliefs and hypotheses while giving disproportionately less attention to alternative possibilities (Kerstholt et al., 2010). Confirmation bias inclines an individual to examine ideas in a one-sided manner, focusing on one possibility and disregarding alternatives, which may ultimately lead to a polarization in beliefs (Jonas, Schulz-Hardt, Frey, & Thelen, 2001; Kassin, Dror, & Kukucka, 2013). Therefore, not only are our negative beliefs more powerful, but we have a bias toward expecting the same outcome time after time. In the event of pervasive relational trauma in childhood, such as rejection, humiliation, or neglect, an individual can develop beliefs that they are unworthy of love and that all people are untrustworthy or abusive. This belief system changes the way an individual perceives themselves and others, in addition to adversely impacting how safe and secure one feels in navigating the world around them.

The Bite That Fits the Wound

When you take a step back and look at your life, you will notice particular patterns and themes that emerge in behaviors, relationships, and even pervasive struggles you encounter. These pervasive patterns are driven by perceptions and choices, which in turn are influenced by the belief system and by the tendency we all have to elevate our belief system when analyzing the world around us. This tendency, known as confirmation bias, inclines an individual to examine ideas in a one-sided manner, focusing on one possibility and disregarding alternatives, which may ultimately lead to a polarization in beliefs. In simple terms, we are hardwired to expect the worst and for history to repeat itself.

The psychological phenomenon of one's inclination to reenact traumatic events and their circumstances has been termed "repetition compulsion" (Freud, 1914). Repetition compulsion is attributed to our predisposition to feel comfortable in the familiar, in addition to the desire to return to an earlier state of things, which in turn can be driven by a desire to rewrite the past. Unconsciously drifting to the familiar is driven by a reparation fantasy, a desire to triumph over the pain experienced at an earlier time (Freud, 1914). Freud's repetition compulsion concept resonates with the human experience of comfort in familiarity and the colloquial concept of "the devil you know." It has been said that if everyone sat in a circle and threw their problems in the middle, with instructions that we could take anyone's problems instead of our own, we all would run and grab our own because they are familiar; we know how they go. We have a desire to solve them and triumph over them. The reparation fantasy lies in the hope that this triumph will render early trauma null and void. A fantasy that does not come true but we continue to chase it nonetheless. As Freud said, we repeat rather than remember.

Unfortunately, the compulsion to repeat past patterns can cause retraumatization and further shame for the trauma survivor. This repeated pattern of relational trauma reenactment has been referred to as "the bite that fits the wound" (Takin & Hendrix, 2011) and points to how the experience of attachment-based relational trauma in the formative years creates a vulnerability to severe emotional dysregulation along with intense feelings of despair, anxiety, shame, and mistrust of others later on in life. This becomes apparent when we see the cycle of abuse. Prisoners of childhood abuse become prisoners of painful or unhealthy relationships in adulthood (Bakermans-Kranenburg & van IJzendoorn, 1997; Mair, Cunradi, & Todd, 2012; Ponti & Tani, 2019). In a more subtle manifestation, when an individual experiences adverse life events in the formative years, they develop a negative self-belief (O'Shea Brown, 2021; Slavich & Auerbach, 2018). This negative belief remains dormant until an individual experiences a traumatic life event that is reminiscent of the original stressor, at which point the preexisting schema or vulnerability becomes activated as a core negative belief (Slavich & Auerbach, 2018).

The case of Rodney[1] illustrates how a 46-year-old gay male encounters a pervasive core negative belief impacting all areas of his life. Rodney is a successful banker, married with two children. He lives with hypertension and hyperglycemia alongside generalized anxiety and panic disorder. Rodney presented to treatment to deal with his panic disorder, which had resulted in him becoming depressed, unmotivated, and deeply dissatisfied with all areas of his life. Rodney expressed that he often felt taken advantage of at work by his boss, colleagues, and even subordinates. From his childhood, he learned to be accommodating and approval seeking and to avoid conflict at all costs. At work this meant that he assumed responsibility for duties that others would normally do and found it difficult to delegate tasks and to set adequate boundaries. Rodney disclosed that his father was physically and emotionally abusive. He expressed that his mother had a warm demeanor; however, in retrospect, he can see that she was submissive to his abusive father.

Rodney lamented that his mother would minimize his hurt and pain as a means of pledging loyalty to his father. This synthesized in a painful memory from adolescence where his father punched him in the face and remarked to Rodney's mother, "He is so selfish that he should go kill himself." This rageful outburst occurred when Rodney returned home 30 min past curfew. Rodney revealed that his father's outbursts were often fleeting, sharp, and grossly disproportionate to the stimuli. Rodney spent much of his childhood walking on eggshells. There was never any apology nor reflective conversations with either parent about the emotional and physical abuse. Instead Rodney's mother would offer him candy, but no words. She never acknowledged his pain, never intervened, and only ever accommodated his father's abuse. As a means of survival through adaptation in an adversarial environment, Rodney became deeply silent, pathologically accommodating, and shame-filled. He learned that he could never set boundaries or advocate for himself.

Consequently, Rodney adopted the core negative belief of "I don't matter." He also learned to self-soothe with food, which he found to be more stable, predictable, and reliable than the people in his life. The central negative cognition – "I don't matter" – remained with him as he was bullied in the school yard for being overweight, taken advantage of at work, and later formed romantic partnerships with controlling, abusive men. Old feelings of exploitation, terror, and sadness haunted him, and he never felt safe or comfortable voicing frustration or making choices based on of his own needs. The core negative belief that he did not matter caused him to feel like a prisoner in all areas of his life. By becoming aware of old patterns of belief and their sources, he was able to begin to challenge his internal dialogue and negative schemas.

The link between core negative beliefs and memories will now be explored, in addition to the method of mapping this connection in a clinical setting.

[1] A pseudonym has been used to preserve confidentiality.

Linking Blocking Beliefs to Memories

In this case illustration, we see how a core negative belief can become a block in the way of wellness and healing. The more that this belief is reinforced and affirmed by one's environment, the more intertwined it can become with one's identity and expression. However, no child is born believing they are unworthy of love, respect, or comfort. This core negative belief is learned through painful experiences and reinforced over time. Core negative beliefs can be viewed as the common threads that are held together and reinforced by traumatic or activating memories (Shapiro, 2018). Sometimes people will have many different core negative beliefs. When you listen closely to a client, you can begin to hear recurring themes and belief systems. Sometimes this will be revealed through very clear "I am" statements. At times, it is a little more ambiguous and difficult to identify. Particular questions will help you to identify the core negative belief.

Finding the Memories Connected to the Core Negative Belief

The following excerpt illustrates the kinds of questions a clinician asked Rodney as part of the process of identifying his core negative belief(s).

Rodney: My parents unfavorably compared me to my brother. This was especially apparent when we would get our report cards and our parents would sit us down for comparison.

Clinician: What is the negative belief that you had about yourself in that moment?

Rodney: "I am ashamed. I will never be like my brother."

Clinician: What does that belief say about you?

Rodney: It says, "I am not good enough."

Clinician: Has that belief been with you throughout your life?

Rodney: Yes, that belief has always been with me.

Clinician: (Writes "I am not good enough" on a piece of paper, and draws a timeline underneath, as shown in Figure 10.) Rodney, I want to invite you to write down 3–5 times in your life when you were made to feel not good enough. You might just write enough to pull the memory from your internal filing cabinet, as if you were reading the headline of a newspaper.

As illustrated in Fig. 7.1, the core negative belief – in this case, "I am not good enough" – is written on the top of a page. Underneath we see how the client has connected the core negative belief with specific memories. The memories serve as an indicator or reminder of how such messages became internalized into the unconscious during the formative years (Shapiro, 2018). Through introspection and reflection, the client can begin to operate out of deep self-awareness rather than classic conditioning. These memories can begin to be processed and targeted through trauma-informed techniques such as Eye Movement Desensitization and

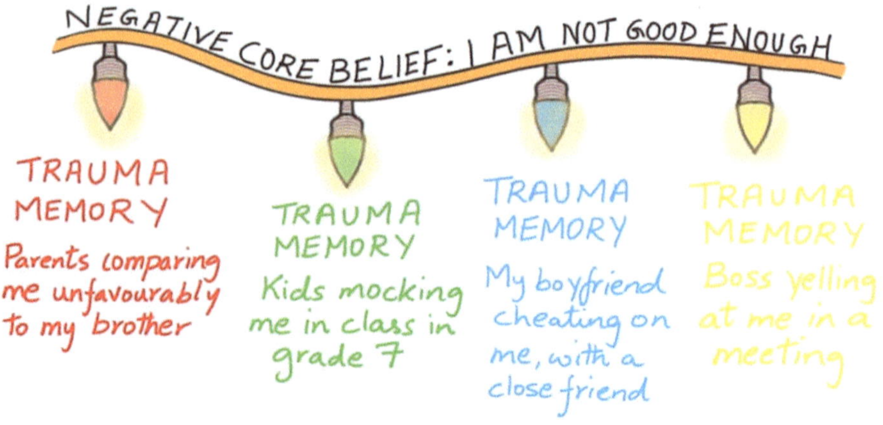

Fig. 7.1 Belief systems and associated memories (Credit: Illustration sourced by EMDR-trained Psychotherapist © Ayan Mukherjee – therapyillustrated.com, used with permission). Ayan Mukherjee is a registered psychotherapist and EMDRIA-approved certified EMDR therapist and Consultant-in-Training, with a private practice in Toronto, Canada. Mukherjee is the creator of the illustrations on Polyvagal Theory and EMDR Reprocessing Phase that have been used in this book. For more information about visual aid tools for trauma therapy: www.TherapyIllustrated.com

Reprocessing or Trauma-Focused Cognitive Behavioral Therapy (as discussed in Chap. 8).

After this exercise, a client can sometimes feel activated or a little exposed. It can be stabilizing under these circumstances to create a more affirming map of positive self-beliefs. This can be done by asking, "Now that you have mapped out your negative core beliefs, what is the belief that you would like to have about yourself?" The client is invited to offer a positive cognition, such as "I am good enough as I am." They will then be directed to repeat the exercise by naming 3–5 moments in their life when they felt "good enough" as they were. This can be challenging for the client; they may need support and guidance in being reminded of any previously discussed sources of pride or contentment. A helpful guiding question during this time is, "When do you feel most yourself?" Even if an individual did not grow up in an environment which made them feel worthwhile and valuable, they may have had some experiences with coworkers, in the community, or even in the therapy room where they learned that their emotions are important and can be expressed safely. This can also be a wonderful opportunity to provide psychoeducation on negativity bias and confirmation bias.

For other clients with more intense somatization, the sensations of the body can be used as a gateway to access cognition and memory. For instance, the client who experiences a tightness in the throat during public speaking may associate this physical sensation with the core negative concept, "I am stupid." When asked to name an earlier memory involving this sensation, they recall the previous experience of floundering over words at a spelling bee. Even though this memory is not readily available in the conscious mind, the implicit memory provides a somatic cue anytime that person is at risk of feeling inadequate or imprudent.

When exploring painful material, it is important to "invite" the client to engage in reflections, to ask their consent before moving forward, and to gauge their comfort level as the discussion progresses (even after they have consented). Self-determination can be promoted throughout the therapeutic relationship, resulting in clients having more choices about their sessions, their boundaries, and their comfort level so that therapeutic goals are agreed upon (Marsh, Angell, Andrews, & Curry, 2012). There is a growing body of evidence, both in health care and mental health care, suggesting that increasing choice promotes positive outcomes, as shared decision-making creates increased satisfaction and improved social functioning (Davidson, 2006; Stanhope, Barrenger, Salzer, & Marcus, 2013). The client must believe that they have power and control over their healing process, in addition to believing that their voice and opinions are of the utmost importance. In this way, the client can become an agent of change in their own life. Meaningful collaboration in cocreating the therapy experience is particularly vital when working with survivors of complex trauma who often feel disempowered due to prolonged relational abuse, neglect, and oppression (Davidson, 2006; Marsh et al., 2012; Stanhope et al., 2013). This is mainly due to past histories of broken promises, boundary violations and intrusions which can later impact the therapeutic alliance. (O'Shea Brown, 2021). Building trust and engagement in the clinical dyad is a delicate process of seeking consent and gauging comfort. The most important component of the therapeutic alliance is the level of trust and comfort level between the client and their clinician. In a synergistic way, if the client can self-advocate, make choices, and set boundaries in the clinical relationship, they can begin to feel more comfort applying these same skills in other areas of their life.

Summary

Our belief system informs our perception of reality, our choices, and our experiences of the world. Beliefs become stronger and even more deeply rooted when they are repeatedly affirmed by our environment. The exploration of core negative belief systems deepens the clinician's understanding of an individual's emotional map by accessing their unconscious drives and motives. It allows you as the clinician to attune sensitively to painful memories, recurring triggers, and blocking belief systems and biases associated with complex relational trauma. A bias is a tendency or inclination toward a particular belief system; some biases can be positive and helpful, and others may cause harm (Munroe et al., 1997). Negativity bias is the principle that "negative events are more salient, potent, dominant in combinations, and generally efficacious than positive events" (Rozin & Royzman, 2001, p. 297). Confirmation bias, meanwhile, inclines the individual to examine ideas in a one-sided manner, focusing on one possibility and disregarding alternatives, which may ultimately lead to a polarization in beliefs (Jonas et al., 2001; Kassin et al., 2013). When working with clients with a history of pervasive relational trauma in childhood characterized by abuse, rejection, humiliation, or neglect, it is important to remember that they may be very doubtful of positive outcomes and trustworthy relationships. Self-determination and the therapeutic alliance have repeatedly been shown to greatly enhance the efficacy of psychotherapy treatment across all modalities (Davidson, 2006; Marsh et al., 2012; Stanhope et al., 2013). Therefore, guiding the client to be more introspective and reflective regarding their belief patterns can create a sense of agency and empowerment. The subsequent chapter shall explore evidence-based modalities used to treat complex trauma.

Questions and Activities for Discussion and Further Reflection

1. Do you understand the terms (i) negative core belief, (ii) negativity bias, and (iii) confirmation bias?
2. Choose two core beliefs (from Table 7.1), one positive and one negative, and complete a timeline connecting them to your own memories (as seen in Fig. 7.1).

Exercise

1. Class Discussion Prompt: Reflect on the narrative of your formative years and life experience today. How have your specific experiences shaped and informed your belief systems?

References

Bakermans-Kranenburg, M. J., & van IJzendoorn, M. H. (1997). Adult attachment and the break-up of romantic relationships. *Journal of Divorce and Remarriage, 27*, 121–139.

Bowlby, J. (1980). *Attachment and loss, III: Loss, sadness, and depression*. New York, NY: Basic Books.

Bowlby, J. (1989). The role of attachment in personality development and psychopathology. In S. I. Greenspan & G. H. Pollack (Eds.), *The course of life: Vol. 1. Infancy* (pp. 119–136). Madison, CT: International Universities Press.

Cacioppo, J. T., Cacioppo, S., & Gollan, J. K. (2014). The negativity bias: Conceptualization, quantification, and individual differences. *Behavioral and Brain Sciences, 37*(3), 309–310. https://doi.org/10.1017/S0140525X13002537

Davidson, L. (2006). The top ten concerns about recovery encountered in mental health system transformation. *Psychiatric Services, 57*, 640–645. https://doi.org/10.1176/appi.ps.57.5.640

Fairbairn, W. R. D. (1943). The repression and the return of bad objects (with special reference to the 'war neuroses'). *British Journal of Medical Psychology, 19*, 327–341. https://doi.org/10.1111/j.2044-8341.1943.tb00328.x

Freud, S. (1914). *Remembering, repeating and working-through (further recommendations on the technique of psycho-analysis II)*. The standard Edition of the Complete Psychological Works of Sigmund Freud, Volume XII (1911–1913): The Case of Schreber, Papers on Technique and Other Works, pp. 145–156.

Jonas, E., Schulz-Hardt, S., Frey, S., & Thelen, N. (2001). Confirmation bias in sequential information search after preliminary decisions: An expansion of dissonance theoretical research on selective exposure to information. *Journal of Personality and Social Psychology, 80*(4), 557–571.

Kassin, S. M., Dror, I. E., & Kukucka, J. (2013). The forensic confirmation bias: Problems, perspectives, and proposed solutions. *Journal of Applied Research in Memory and Cognition, 2*(1), 42–52.

Kerstholt, J., Eikelboom, A., Dijkman, T., Stoel, R., Hermsen, R., & van Leuven, B. (2010). Does suggestive information cause a confirmation bias in bullet comparisons? *Forensic Science International, 198*(1–3). https://doi.org/10.1016/j.forsciint.2010.02.007

Kirshner, L. A. (1991). The concept of the self in psychoanalytic theory and its philosophical foundations. *Journal of the American Psychoanalytic Association, 39*(1), 157–182. https://doi.org/10.1177/000306519103900108

Kohut, H. (1977). *The restoration of the self.* University of Chicago Press.

Lee, A., & Hankin, B. L. (2009). Insecure attachment, dysfunctional attitudes, and low self-esteem predicting prospective symptoms of depression and anxiety during adolescence. *Journal of Clinical Child and Adolescent Psychology, 38*, 219–231.

Main, M., & Hesse, E. (1990). Parents' unresolved traumatic experiences are related to infant disorganized attachment status: Is frightened and/or frightening parental behavior the linking mechanism? In M. Greenberg, D. Cichetti, & M. Cummings (Eds.), *Attachment in the preschool years* (pp. 161–182). Chicago, IL: University of Chicago Press Division. 53, 38(2), pp. 219–231. https://doi.org/10.1080/15374410802698396

Mair, C., Cunradi, C. B., & Todd, M. (2012). Adverse childhood experiences and intimate partner violence: Testing psychosocial mediational pathways among couples. *Annals of Epidemiology, 22*(12), 832–839. https://doi.org/10.1016/j.annepidem.2012.09.008

Marsh, J. C., Angell, B., Andrews, C. M., & Curry, A. (2012). Client-provider relationship and treatment outcome: A systematic review of substance abuse, child welfare, and mental health services research. *Journal of the Society for Social Work and Research, 3*, 233–267. https://doi.org/10.5243/jsswr.2012.15

Moseley, J. B., O'Malley, K., Petersen, N. J., Menke, T. J., Brody, B. A., Kuykendall, D. H., … Wray, N. P. (2002). A controlled trial of arthroscopic surgery for osteoarthritis of the knee. *The New England Journal of Medicine, 347*(2), 81–88. Retrieved from http://proxy.library.nyu.edu/login?url=https://search-proquest-com.proxy.library.nyu.edu/docview/223938313?accountid=12768

Munroe, A., Smutzler, N., & Bates, L. (1997). A brief review of the research on husband violence Part III: Sociodemographic factors, relationship factors, and differing consequences of husband and wife violence. *Aggression and Violent Behavior 2*(3), 285–307.

O'Shea Brown, G. (2020). Internal family systems informed eye movement desensitization and reprocessing: An integrative technique for treatment of complex posttraumatic stress disorder. *International Body Psychotherapy Journal, 19*(2), 112–122.

O'Shea Brown, G. (2021). Reflections on providing virtual eye movement desensitization and reprocessing therapy in the wake of COVID-19: Survival through adaptation. In C. Tosone (Ed.), *Shared trauma, Shared resilience during a pandemic: Social work in the time of COVID-19*. Cham, Switzerland: Springer.

Ponti, L., & Tani, F. (2019). Attachment bonds as risk factors of intimate partner violence. *Journal of Child and Family Studies, 28*(5), 1425–1432. https://doi.org/10.1007/s10826-019-01361-4

Rozin, R., & Royzman, E. B. (2001). Negativity bias, negativity dominance, and contagion. *Personality and Social Psychology Review, 4*, 296–320.

Shapiro, F. (2018). *Eye Movement Desensitization and Reprocessing (EMDR) therapy: Basic principles protocols, and procedures* (3rd ed.). New York, NY: The Guilford Press.

Shapiro, F., & Forrest, M. S. (2016). *EMDR: Breakthrough therapy for overcoming anxiety, stress & trauma*. New York, NY: Basic Books.

Slavich, G. M., & Auerbach, R. P. (2018). Stress and its sequelae: Depression, suicide, inflammation, and physical illness. In J. N. Butcher & J. M. Hooley (Eds.), *APA handbook of psy-*

chopathology, Vol. 1: Psychopathology: Understanding, assessing, and treating adult mental disorders (pp. 375–402). Washington, DC: American Psychological Association.

Stanhope, V., Barrenger, S. L., Salzer, M. S., & Marcus, S. C. (2013). Examining the relationship between choice, therapeutic Alliance and outcomes in mental health services. *Journal of Personalized Medicine, 3*(3), 191–202. https://doi.org/10.3390/jpm3030191

Takin, S., & Hendrix, H. (2011). *Wired for love: How understanding your partner's brain and attachment style can help you defuse conflict and build a secure relationship*. CA: New Harbinger Publications.

van IJzendoorn, M. H. (1995). Adult attachment representations, parental responsiveness, and infant attachment: A meta-analysis on the predictive validity of the Adult Attachment Interview. *Psychological Bulletin, 117*, 387–403.

Chapter 8
An Overview of Psychotherapy Modalities for the Treatment of Complex Trauma

The term "complex trauma" is used to describe chronic traumatization, for instance, the experience of multiple and/or prolonged, developmentally adverse traumatic events, most often of an interpersonal nature. Complex trauma is the result of chronic, prolonged, and repeated trauma arising from childhood abuse, neglect, and/or exposure to domestic violence (Herman, 1992; van der Kolk, McFarlane, & Weisaeth, 1996). The field of psychotherapy has increasingly become influenced by evidence-based practice (EBP), which is centered on the ethos of research-informed practice and practice-informed research (Drisko & Grady, 2019). Consequently, treatment planning and the clinical decision-making process are informed by best practice guidelines developed from research findings. Research has consistently shown that the treatment of complex trauma should be phase-oriented, multimodal, and skill-focused, with a core emphasis on symptom relief and functional improvement (Briere & Scott, 2006; Courtois, Ford, & Cloitre, 2009; van der Kolk, 2015).

Within this holistic, integrative framework, there is an appreciation of the mind-body connection. Complex trauma treatment has evolved into a more integrative, body-oriented approach. This chapter provides an overview of complex trauma treatments, including Trauma-Focused Cognitive Behavioral Therapy (TF-CBT), Eye Movement Desensitization and Reprocessing (EMDR), and other body-based modalities such as Sensorimotor Psychotherapy (SP) and Somatic Experiencing (SE); however, this does not serve as a substitute for the necessary training(s). Please see the Appendix for information on training(s).

This chapter will first provide an overview of Trauma-Focused Cognitive Behavioral Therapy as a psychotherapy modality for treating complex trauma. Second, an outline of the process of Eye Movement Desensitization and Reprocessing therapy will be offered. Subsequently, a review of the benefit of body-based therapies such as Sensorimotor Psychotherapy and Somatic Experiencing shall be discussed. Finally, this chapter shall discuss the implications for somatic therapies arising from COVID-19—more specifically, the fact that virtual therapy has gone from being an emerging trend in clinical practice to a necessary adaptation during COVID-19.

G. O'Shea Brown, *Healing Complex Posttraumatic Stress Disorder*, Essential Clinical Social Work Series, https://doi.org/10.1007/978-3-030-61416-4_8

Trauma-Focused Cognitive Behavioral Therapy

The efficacy of Trauma-Focused Cognitive Behavioral Therapy (TF-CBT) has been well established, with a large evidence base of randomized trials supporting its use in the treatment of trauma and complex trauma (Cohen, Deblinger, Mannarino, & Steer, 2004; Cohen, Mannarino, & Deblinger, 2006; Cohen, Mannarino, & Knudsen, 2005; Deblinger, Mannarino, Cohen, & Steer, 2006; Jensen et al., 2014). TF-CBT is a skills-based modality used to treat child, adolescent, and adult survivors of trauma, which combines techniques of cognitive behavioral therapy and family therapy. It was first developed in the 1990s by Judith Cohen, MD; Esther Deblinger, PhD; and Anthony Mannarino, PhD, as a modality designed to reduce trauma-related symptomatology. The objective of TF-CBT is to foster the growth of adaptive skills and communication techniques outside of the therapy suite. TF-CBT can be administered in the context of individual and/or family therapy counseling sessions; most commonly there is an interweave of the two (Cohen et al., 2006). As TF-CBT is a skills-based model, and when applied to a family therapy scenario it requires the child and parent to practice its components in order to be optimally effective, clients are often asked to practice skills at home. This creates a sense of empowerment, resiliency, and self-determination within the therapeutic process. TF-CBT treatment is specifically tailored to meet the needs of the individual or the family and is centered upon core concepts which include psychoeducation, parenting skills, affect regulation, cognitive processing of traumatic/painful material, and formulating a trauma narrative, in addition to enhancing future safety (Cohen et al., 2004, 2005; Deblinger et al., 2006).

In the beginning phases of TF-CBT, psychoeducation about the impacts of trauma can be very helpful in facilitating the survivor to process their emotions and understand their physiological responses to activating stimuli. The TF-CBT model hypothesizes that the fear of being threatened or at risk of harm evokes a physiological response that prompts the body to activate responses related to trauma (Bisson, 2009). Exposure to trauma can lead to cognitive distortions in the areas of safety, trust, and self-concept, in addition to avoidance of thoughts, feelings, or reminders of the trauma (American Psychiatric Association, 2013). TF-CBT skills teach the survivor how to better manage emotional responses and behavioral patterns related to the trauma by facilitating cognitive restructuring of trauma-related memories with the goal of reducing, and eventually eliminating, trauma-related symptoms (Lanius et al., 2010). This can often occur through reflective questioning or workbook exercises. As illustrated in Table 8.1, the client is usually asked to measure the benefits versus the drawbacks of avoiding versus facing a trauma trigger.

By gently navigating which side of this diagram has more "pros" than "cons," the client can begin to feel empowered to make an informed decision while also appraising the impulse to avoid. This guided introspection can be a very effective way of understanding behavioral patterns and thought processes compassionately. In a typical TF-CBT intervention, the client is guided through confronting the disturbing event in addition to being provided with psychoeducation, exposure, cognitive restructuring, and affect management training (Harvey, Bryant, & Tarrier, 2003). Furthermore, cognitive behavioral techniques are employed to modify mal-

Table 8.1 An example of a TF-CBT thought exercise: navigating the challenges of unhealthy family relationships where estrangement feels like too much but boundaries are necessary for safety and healing

Avoidance	Facing the trauma/fear
Benefits: If I avoid going home I know won't be yelled at, called names and made to feel shameful. This feels safer to me.	Benefits: If I go to see my mother I will feel less guilty and disconnected from the family system.
Risks: By not going home I will feel like I am a bad person. I know that I will feel guilty and shameful for several months afterwards.	Risks: By visiting her, it is highly likely that I will be yelled at and called pejorative names. I could be retraumatized given what has happened repeatedly in the past. The only way to limit this risk is to visit for a short period of time, to rent a car and have somewhere to stay outside of the home.

adaptive thought processes and negative reactive behaviors in a trauma-informed manner. Examples of this may include acknowledging emotions, understanding their triggers, reframing the narrative, and co-creating plans to ensure future safety. Information on training and certification is provided in the Appendix.

Eye Movement Desensitization and Reprocessing

Eye Movement Desensitization and Reprocessing is a therapy modality designed to resolve unprocessed traumatic memories in the body and nervous system, created by Francine Shapiro, PhD, in the 1980s. The efficacy of EMDR therapy in the treatment of PTSD has been well established, as evidenced by the results of over 30 positive randomized controlled studies over the past three decades (Ahmad, Larsson, & Sundelin-Wahlsten, 2007; Chen et al., 2018; Marcus, Marquis, & Sakai, 2004; Wilson, Becker, & Tinker, 1997). Such findings led the World Health Organization (2013) to state that TF-CBT and EMDR are the only psychotherapy modalities recommended in the treatment of children, adolescents, and adults who meet the diagnostic criteria for PTSD. It is important to note that most of the randomized controlled study participants differ from survivors of complex trauma with chronic abuse and neglect histories in terms of symptom presentation and capacity for tolerating trauma-focused work (Korn, 2009). Many of the participants presented to therapy seeking treatment for single incident trauma rather than for complex trauma. The treatment of complex trauma should be phase-oriented, multimodal, and skill-focused, with a core emphasis on symptom relief and functional improvement (Briere & Scott, 2006; Courtois et al., 2009; van der Kolk, 2015). This multi-phased skill-based model prompts reflection and mindfulness, which, in turn, allows the client to operate out of deep self-awareness rather than conditioning.

EMDR incorporates the Adaptive Information Processing (AIP) model, which posits that memories of distressing experiences are dysfunctionally stored in the brain in an unmetabolized state in the memory networks that contain perceptions, negative beliefs, affective states, and body sensations that arose during the trauma experience (Shapiro, 2007). When memories are stored this way, the brain, much like a "skipping disc," will replay the most distressing parts of the memory over and over, causing intrusive thoughts, shame-based cognition, and psychological reactivity that can be activated by sensitivity cues (Shapiro, 2001). Shapiro (2001) further hypothesized that there is an "innate physiological system that is designed to transform disturbing input into an adaptive resolution and a psychologically healthy integration" (p.54). Since its inception, EMDR has been understood by both clinicians and clients as a powerful vehicle for processing traumatic experience, but one to be undertaken only when the client has achieved stabilization (Shapiro, 1989, 1991).

EMDR involves eight phases, which include the following steps: (1) history-taking; (2) preparation and stabilization; (3) assessment; (4–7) desensitization, reprocessing, and closure; and finally (8) reevaluation (Shapiro, 1995). This multi-phased protocol is illustrated in Fig. 8.1. The foundation of EMDR treatment involves providing the client with psychoeducation around dissociation and trauma processing, in addition to teaching affect regulation techniques. The preparatory steps involve history-taking and stabilization, and the client is encouraged to employ affect regulation techniques (known as positive resourcing) autonomously, both within and outside of the therapy room. During this preparatory phase of treatment, there is a strong emphasis on building affect tolerance (a sense of safety in the body) and psychoeducation. These efforts are known as Resource Development and Installation (RDI).

Leeds (1995) introduced RDI, along with proposed principles for the use of bilateral stimulation along with positive images and memories. RDI was incorporated into the EMDR protocol early on and has been utilized to strengthen affective, cognitive, and behavioral coping skills (Korn & Leeds, 2002; Shapiro, 1995). EMDR-RDI refers to a set of EMDR protocols which focus exclusively on strengthening connections to positive affective states and resourceful memories (Korn & Leeds, 2002; Leeds, 1995; Leeds & Shapiro, 2000). EMDR-RDI is used to help clients access existing resources and develop new and effective coping skills, such as mindfulness, self-soothing, distancing, containment, titration, grounding, and emotional regulation (Leeds & Shapiro, 2000). EMDR-RDI focuses on stabilizing and preparing clients for the next phases of treatment, when attention will turn to the processing of traumatic memories (O'Shea Brown 2021). A central feature of complex trauma is a loss of the ability to physiologically modulate stress responses in addition to a diminished capacity to utilize bodily signals (van der Kolk et al., 1996). EMDR-RDI can be very effective in increasing affect tolerance when it is used to enhance mindfulness, the ability to notice a feeling or bodily sensation and accompanying emotions (Korn, 2009). Survivors of complex trauma often present with increased dissociative symptoms; therefore, establishing safety in the body is paramount to the healing process (Forgash & Copeley, 2008). The efficacy of EMDR can be challenged by symptoms of dissociation and complex trauma; therefore, RDI is highly beneficial to the efficacy of treatment (Fisher, 2002; Korn & Leeds, 2002).

Once stabilization has been established, the client and clinician can begin to agree on "target memories" to be processed. EMDR is a trauma resolution approach that involves a standard set of procedures and clinical protocols to determine the target memories, and these protocols include specific types of bilateral sensory

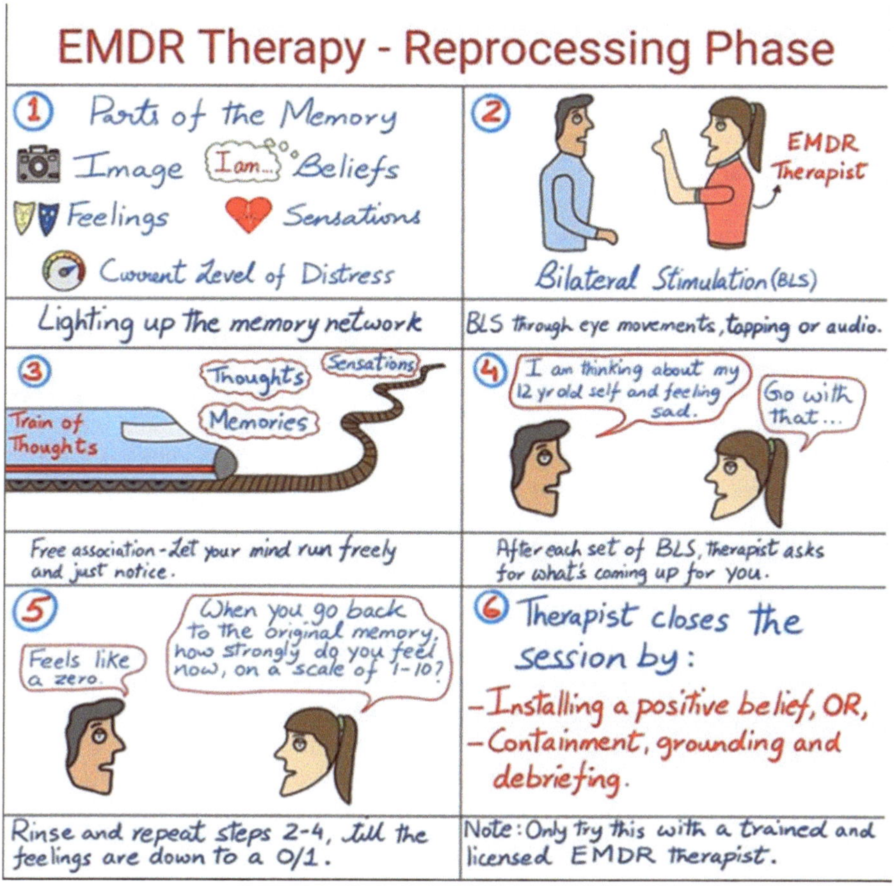

Fig. 8.1 EMDR therapy – reprocessing stage (Credit: Illustration sourced by EMDR-trained Psychotherapist © Ayan Mukherjee – therapyillustrated.com, used with permission). Ayan Mukherjee is a registered psychotherapist and EMDRIA-approved certified EMDR therapist and Consultant-in-Training, with a private practice in Toronto, Canada. Mukherjee is the creator of the illustrations on Polyvagal Theory and EMDR Reprocessing Phase that have been used in this book. For more information about visual aid tools for trauma therapy: www.TherapyIllustrated.com

stimulation. Bilateral stimulation is the use of visual, auditory, or tactile external stimuli presented in a rhythmic and/or side-to-side pattern. This is determined by the individuals' expressed preference and comfort level. Once the clinician and the client have agreed upon which memory to target, the client is asked to hold different aspects of the event in their mind, while bilateral stimulation is occurring. The bilateral stimulation can occur through bilateral eye movements guided by the clinician's hand, a therapulse, tapping, or through auditory stimulation (alternate tone to the left and right ear) based on the client's comfort or preference.

As this happens, for reasons believed by Robert Stickgold, PhD, a neurobiological researcher at Harvard Medical School, to be connected with the biological mechanisms involved in rapid eye movement (REM) sleep, internal associations arise, enabling the client to begin processing the target memory and disturbing feelings that accompany it. Stickgold (2002) proposed that the repetitive bilateral stimulation in EMDR induces a neurobiological state similar to the REM of restful sleep and hypothesized that this state supports the cortical integration of traumatic memories into general semantic networks. In simple terms, memories can be fully processed through EMDR, along with the painful, distressing stimuli which accompany them.

The specific focused strategies of EMDR along with the bilateral stimulation help access the client's dysfunctionally stored memories and related affect, which in turn desensitizes the emotions and physical sensations associated with the traumatic memory, enabling the client to access more adaptive material stored in the brain and forge new, more positive associations with the original event. In successful EMDR therapy, the meaning of painful events is transformed on an emotional level. For instance, a rape victim shifts from feeling horror and self-disgust to holding the firm belief that "The trauma has passed and now I am safe" or "It was not my fault; I am a good person." EMDR activates a healing process in many clients where scenes from the past are witnessed compassionately and often inner child parts of self are unburdened from guilt and shame (O'Shea Brown, 2020; Twombly & Schwartz, 2008). Among EMDR-trained clinicians, there are an acknowledgment of the presence of an innate physiological healing system and thus an acknowledgment that the insights clients gain in EMDR therapy result not so much from clinician interpretation, but from their own accelerated intellectual and emotional processes. Information on training and certification is provided in the Appendix.

Case Study

The following case study is a composite case which contains elements and techniques derived from a number of EMDR sessions. Kate[1] is a 36-year-old married Caucasian female, employed full-time in health care. Kate has a diagnosis of complex posttraumatic stress disorder and presented to treatment with symptoms of shame based cognition and intrusive thoughts due to a history of relational trauma including child physical abuse and emotional abuse. Over the course of her treatment thus far, history-taking has revealed pervasive negative cognition, including pervasive thoughts of weakness and inadequacy. Kate reported repeated disturbing memories, somatic symptoms related to trauma, pervasive guilt, low mood, and hypervigilance arising from childhood complex trauma. The following excerpt illustrates the process of Kate being guided through the installation of a "relational resource" (Korn and Leeds, 2002) as adapted from Fisher's Modified EMDR-RDI Protocol (Fisher, 2001).

[1] A pseudonym has been used to preserve confidentiality.

Clinician: Sit back in the chair, connect with your body and begin to breathe deep into the stomach.
You are seated with your feet on the ground (Pause).
Please think about a place that feels calm (Pause).
When you have the image of what represents your calm place, I want you to let me know by nodding.
Kate: (nods).
Clinician: Tell me what you see.
Kate: I am sitting in the garden. It has a beautiful patio. It's a warm day and I feel peaceful.
Clinician: As you think of that experience notice what you see, hear and feel.
Notice what emotions you are experiencing and how you feel in your body (6–8 Sets Bilateral Stimulation).
Kate: My body feels calm. I see lush green grass…the sky is blue and my skin is warm from the sun.
Clinician: Notice that….
Kate: The air is cool. I feel calm. It is peaceful up here.
I feel connected to my body. I feel like I can breathe easily up here.
My body feels lighter and looser.
Clinician: Focus on your calm place and its sights, sounds, smells, and sensations (Pause). Tell me more about your experience (6–8 Sets Bilateral Stimulation).
Kate: I can see the patio clearly. The greenery looks so beautiful and I hear the leaves move in the wind. The air is cool and fresh. I am enjoying the view.
My shoulders are loose and I am breathing deeply and easily.
Clinician: Bring up the current image (Pause).
Concentrate on where you feel the pleasant sensations in your body and allow yourself to enjoy them. Concentrate on those sensations. (6–8 Sets Bilateral Stimulation).
Kate: (shoulders drop, jaw is unclenched, client has a slight grin).
Clinician: What are you noticing now? (6–8 Sets Bilateral Stimulation).
Kate: Cool and fresh air and the gentle movement of the leaves.
There is no chaos up here, only harmony.
My body is rested. I feel the warmth of the sun on my skin.
Clinician: Focus on that. What do you notice now? (6–8 Sets Bilateral Stimulation).
Kate: I feel calm in my body. I feel it in my stomach. It feels peaceful.
Clinician: Is there a word or phrase that represents your calm place? (6–8 Sets Bilateral Stimulation).
Kate: Serenity.
Clinician: Think of the word 'serenity' and notice the positive feelings and sensations you are having when you think of that word (substantial pause).
Concentrate on those sensations and the word 'serenity' and be curious about the sensation.
What are you noticing now? (6–8 Sets Bilateral Stimulation).
Kate: My heart feels warm and I feel safe.

Clinician: Now, place your hand on your heart center and say the word 'serenity' and notice how you feel. (6–8 Sets Bilateral Stimulation).

Kate: I feel strong and powerful (grins).

Clinician: Allow that word to metabolize in your body. (Pause).

Ok, wonderful, come back again to the room. Gently come back to your body and open your eyes.

Kate: I am here, I feel anchored.

Clinician: You did wonderfully.

We need to find a way to support you in processing painful material.

What inner strength or resource would help you feel less overwhelmed?

Kate: I feel like I am always alone when I am most vulnerable. It scares me when people lose control and become unpredictable and hurtful.

Clinician: Is there a reliable, nurturing figure that could serve as a supportive guide to you?

Kate: My friend Caroline[2] would always listen to me and find a way to make me feel important. She is so kind, the way she looks at me – there is a warmth that surrounds her.

Clinician: That is a wonderful choice for a warm nurturing figure. I could hear the warmth in your voice as you recalled her warm nurturing presence.

Close your eyes and imagine what it would feel like to have her presence as a resource (6–8 Sets Bilateral Stimulation).

Kate: I would feel safe and special. I know I matter to her.

She makes me feel safe.

Clinician: Yes, and if you felt safer, what would follow from that? (6–8 Sets Bilateral Stimulation).

Kate: I feel safe and special.

Clinician: Once again, imagine yourself with Caroline, imagine her warm presence and gentle smile. In every cell of your body, you feel safer and even more protected.

(Pause).

Notice the feeling in your body that goes with having a warm nurturing figure available to you. (6–8 Sets Bilateral Stimulation).

Kate: My throat is open; stomach feels neutral.

I feel very connected to her right now.

Clinician: Yes, with Caroline available to you, you feel calmer and more peaceful —go with that. (6–8 Sets Bilateral Stimulation).

Kate: (smiling) (hands are placed on heart center).

Clinician: What would Caroline say to that sensation? (6–8 Sets Bilateral Stimulation).

Kate: You are here and you are safe.

Clinician: You are here and you are safe.

---

[2] A pseudonym has been used to preserve confidentiality.

Slowly, slowly come back into this room, noticing your toes in your shoes, tongue in your mouth, eyes fluttering and when you're ready I want you to reenter the room.

How are you feeling, Kate? (6–8 Sets Bilateral Stimulation).

Kate: I feel safe and connected. I am never alone.

Clinician: Yes. You are here and you are safe. Your warm nurturing figure will be available to you whenever you need to call upon her as we embark further on your healing journey.

Despite its structured protocol, EMDR therapy remains a highly relational process. The foundational steps of EMDR processing involve providing the client with psychoeducation around dissociation, trauma, and affect regulation techniques. EMDR clinicians must have the clinical awareness to know when to provide therapeutic assistance for grounding and restabilizing (O'Shea Brown 2021; Watson-Wong, 2013). It is critical for therapists to build strong attunement and communication skills to ensure optimal connection with the client during EMDR. EMDR is designed to be a gentle relational process. After an initial phase of establishing safety in the body and mapping out history, the focus is on compassionate witnessing of trauma. EMDR activates a healing process in many clients, where scenes from the past are witnessed compassionately and often inner child parts of self are unburdened from guilt and shame (O'Shea Brown, 2020). During EMDR, the client has one foot in the present and one foot in the past as they are guided to process past events. This dual awareness is an important part of the processing, as a client never feels completely "in" the pain—rather, they are witnessing it from a point of safety. Trauma, when it occurs, is often fast and painful, and in contrast EMDR treatment can feel slow and gentle, with the client connecting with their own innate wisdom and power as a mechanism of healing.

Sensorimotor Psychotherapy

Research has found a strong correlation between affect dysregulation and early complex trauma, neglect, and/or attachment failure (Courtois, Ford, & Cloitre, 2009; Ford, Courtois, Steele, van der Hart, & Nijenhuis, 2005; Siegel, 1999; van der Kolk, 2015). In the absence of adequate regulation of infant distress states, Schore (2003) postulates that the development of autonomic nervous system and affect-regulating brain structures are adversely impacted. In the treatment of complex trauma, maladaptive defenses need to be relinquished as new coping skills, self-capacities, and resources are developed and strengthened (Korn, 2009). There are times when TF-CBT and EMDR can feel overwhelming to the trauma survivor (Fisher, 2001; Fisher, 2019). There are times when words will only get you so far. Body-oriented approaches, such as Sensorimotor Psychotherapy (Ogden, Minton, & Pain, 2006) and Somatic Experiencing (Levine, 1997), offer a range of valuable resourcing interventions and exercises that can be either incorporated into the RDI phase of EMDR treatment or used highly effectively on their own.

Sensorimotor Psychotherapy (SP) was developed in the late 1980s by psychologist Pat Ogden, PhD. The theoretical model of SP is built on traditionally accepted therapeutic interventions and neurologically informed trauma research (Ogden & Fisher, 2006). At the time of this publication, there are no formal randomized controlled studies to measure the efficacy of the modality as a treatment for trauma or complex trauma. Studies by Langmuir, Kirsh, and Classen (2012) and Gene-Cos, Fisher, Ogden, and Cantrell (2016) report decreases in physiological and psychological symptoms following SP treatment; however, more research is needed to substantiate the efficacy of SP in the treatment of trauma and complex trauma.

SP is a somatically oriented talk therapy which approaches affect dysregulation as a subcortical physiological issue central to the treatment of traumatic stress (Ogden, Minton, et al., 2006; Fisher, 2019). As SP does not require the use of touch (hands-on intervention), it is a somatic approach which can be integrated into other therapy modalities for trauma-related disorders (Fisher, 2019). The Sensorimotor Psychotherapy Institute offers progressive levels of training in SP, from beginning (Level 1) through advanced (Level 3) in addition to training in working with clients who present with complex trauma and dissociation. SP works to defuse the dysregulated autonomic arousal and support the client in building resources to manage their emotions and process their trauma safely (Ogden, Pain & Fisher, 2006). SP was developed to address the resolution of somatic symptoms related to unresolved trauma; therefore, bodily experience becomes the primary entry point for intervention, while emotional expression and meaning-making arise out of the subsequent somatic reorganization of habitual trauma-related responses (Ogden, Pain et al., 2006).

Bowlby (1989) hypothesized that a child's earliest experiences with their parents lead to the development of beliefs regarding self-worth, safety, security, and the trustworthiness of others, which he termed the "internal working model." Children make sense of the world by creating emotional maps to assist them in discerning who they should trust and how they will survive. SP is connected to attachment and early relational experiences, which form the internal working model and the somatic narrative. When a trauma is not fully processed, the individual may re-experience the event on a somatic level. This becomes part of the somatic narrative (Ogden & Fisher, 2006). Examples of a somatic narrative for a trauma survivor may include physical pain, numbing, hyperarousal of emotions, or rapid heartbeat. SP connects with bodily sensations as a source of communication, which can increase the flexibility of relational responses, actions, and arousal levels (Ogden & Fisher, 2006). In layman's terms, by understanding the body's responses as a form of internal wisdom or communication, a person can deepen their self-awareness and feel more empowered within their body.

Somatic narratives fall within the scope of implicit memory. Implicit memory describes the process by which past experiences are remembered without conscious effort. One of its common forms is procedural memory. For instance, we access our procedural memory when brushing our teeth, bicycling, and even driving. Actions that rely on implicit memory are supported by previous experiences, classic conditioning, and priming. Regardless of how long ago experiences occurred, individuals can perform the tasks stored as implicit memory without conscious effort. Somatic narratives are created by similar mechanisms in the brain. Masero (2017) explains that there is an innate wisdom of the body by which somatic narratives create "procedurally learned habits" which are then encoded in procedural memory. This imprint can take the form of posture, gestures, physical movement, prosody, and even eye contact. Through the experience of SP, it becomes possible for the trauma survivor to address the more primitive, automatic, and involuntary functions of the brain that underpin the trauma symptoms. This is especially useful in the case of preverbal trauma, that is, trauma that occurred before a survivor fully developed the capacity for language.

After the somatic narrative is compassionately witnessed and understood, SP offers useful interventions to interrupt procedural habits stuck in the past and to enhance the client's abilities to feel safe, seek proximity, and set boundaries within relationships (Masero, 2017). SP is a very useful therapeutic modality for addressing challenges posed by the implicit memory, since it provides access to parts of the self that could not be accessed through language alone (Ogden & Fisher, 2006). By the clinician's compassionately witnessing the client's bodily responses to traumatic material, the client's ability to improve affect regulation is developed; this is a significant benefit of the use of SP. SP treatment is also designed to prevent retraumatization by building resources for the modulation of emotion and arousal. Please see the Appendix for information on training and certification in this modality.

Somatic Experiencing

For many trauma survivors, the body can become a source of pain, shame, or intrusion; therefore, locating safety in the body is one of the foundational steps of trauma treatment. Somatic Experiencing (SE) is a body-focused therapy designed by Peter Levine, PhD, over the past 45 years. SE integrates bodily awareness into the psychotherapeutic process as a means to resolve the symptoms of chronic stress and posttraumatic stress (Levine, 1977). The efficacy of SE has begun to be established through research studies and randomized controlled trials supporting its use in the treatment of trauma, complex trauma, and vicarious trauma (Brom et al., 2017; Parker, Doctor, & Selvam, 2008; Winblad, Changaris, & Stein, 2018). Levine sought to understand how to heal human trauma by observing the autonomic nervous system response of animals under threat in the wild. While both SE and SP track physiological symptoms related to trauma by incorporating the neurobiological model, the two modalities are very distinct with unique objectives. For example, SP techniques are categorized according to various criteria, for instance, whether the trauma is developmental or shock trauma or whether the phase of treatment is stabilization or memory processing. From here SP uses a particular language to link attachment patterns to core beliefs, emotions, and behaviors (Ogden & Fisher, 2006). Rather than focusing on verbal cognitive processes, SE places emphasis on the functioning of the deeper, regulatory levels of the nervous system, in particular the autonomic nervous system, the emotional motor system, the limbic system, and reticular arousal (Payne, Levine, & Crane-Godreau, 2015). SE is a set of techniques and concepts that you can apply to any modality; there are no set protocols.

SE is utilized to create awareness of inner physical sensations, which are seen as the carriers of traumatic memory (Levine, 1997, 2010). Levine (1997) famously said that one of the most painful aspects of trauma is not the event itself but what remains stored inside the trauma survivor in the absence of an empathic witness. Thus, within SE, trauma-related symptomology is not caused by the traumatic event itself, but arises when residual energy from the experience is not discharged from the body (Levine, 1997). When an individual is unable to feel, to express, or to release this energy, it remains internalized and causes long-term dysregulation in the autonomic and central nervous system (Levine, 1977, 1997). The SE approach releases traumatic shock and can be applied to a range of traumatic incidents including drowning, exposure to natural disaster, burns, automobile accidents, and the wounds of emotional and early developmental attachment trauma. SE guides the client's attention to a wide range of internal sensations, including interoceptive (visceral), kinesthetic (musculoskeletal), and proprioceptive experience (Paine et al., 2015). For instance, defensive orienting in the form of hypervigilance, fight, fright, or freeze is more easily triggered in an individual who has been traumatized. Within SE, restoration of healthy and adaptive orienting responses is a critical element in trauma recovery. The trauma survivor is guided in monitoring the body's arousal responses and tracking physiological symptoms through questions such as:

What are you noticing/experiencing right now?
Where do you feel that in your body?
What are the characteristics, sensations, qualities?
Where are you sensing that?
What are you noticing there?

SE broadens a survivor's awareness of their body by eliciting the client's self-report of sensations and other inner experiences, ultimately facilitating a sense of release. SE provides the survivor with the capacity to discharge arousal through learned techniques such as titration, pendulation, resourcing, and managing overcoupling between different elements of experience (Levine, 1997; Payne et al., 2015), for instance, the coupling of feeling physical compression of the chest with feelings of worry or panic or the coupling of intense eye contact with fear. Please see the Appendix for information on training and certification in this modality.

Practice Innovations in the Wake of COVID-19

The spread of the COVID-19 virus has led to severe public health challenges, including detrimental physical and mental health outcomes nationwide. While this is a time of collective trauma, the effects of COVID-19 are undoubtedly giving rise to unequal degrees of hardship, primarily impacting those who are most vulnerable to structural and systemic inequality. The long-term psychological impact of the COVID-19 virus, related both to its spread and to the restrictive policies adopted to counteract it, remains uncertain. However, recent research indicates the pandemic has heightened risk of trauma-related symptoms, which suggests it may exacerbate C-PTSD symptoms for several reasons (Forte, Favieri, Tambelli, & Casagrande, 2020; Zandifar & Badrfam, 2020; Shigemura et al., 2020). Qualitative data from the countries that were among the first to be impacted has shown an increased rate of anxiety, depression, and PTSD, as a some of the psychological consequences of the COVID-19 pandemic (Kang et al., 2020; Tan et al., 2020). A systematic review of 13 studies conducted by Pappa et al. (2020) revealed an increased prevalence in the rate of anxiety by 23.2%, depression by 22.8%, and insomnia by 38.9%.

Social distancing, confinement, and quarantine were adopted to contain diffusion, but these measures have altered the fabric of society, creating changes to consciousness and awakening a climate of trepidation. Many individuals struggled to adapt as strong relational bonds, community ties, and the camaraderie and meaning-making provided by education institutes and places of religious practice were abruptly taken away. This abrupt loss of social norms has the potential to activate hypervigilance in many trauma survivors while also creating a large-scale sense of uncertainty characteristic of a global pandemic (Forte et al., 2020).

The precipitous unfolding of COVID-19 has caused many rapid changes in the provision of psychotherapy; most notably, telepsychotherapy has suddenly become a necessary clinical practice adaptation where it had recently represented an emerging clinical trend. At the time of this publication, there are no randomized controlled trials to measure the efficacy of this transition, and literature on the topic is limited. Telepsychotherapy has grown increasingly more popular over the past two decades and has been recognized as effective for the assessment and diagnosis of many different diverse populations and age groups in various contexts, and from the data, the benefits seem comparable to the face-to-face equivalent (Hilty et al., 2013; Kramer et al., 2012; Langarizadeh et al., 2017). Telepsychotherapy services can be administered in a variety of ways including asynchronous, mobile, and collaborative care and appear to be effectual while increasing the accessibility of care.

EMDR has always been associated with technology, as various devices—such as the pulsars and lightbar—were created to assist with bilateral saccadic eye movements and other forms of sensory dual attention mechanisms. Continued advancement in technology has enhanced the development and utilization of mobile health applications (mHealth apps) using Eye Movement Desensitization and Reprocessing (EMDR) techniques to facilitate the therapeutic process (Shapiro, 2018). However, research measuring the efficacy and safety of these applications is limited, particularly for clients who may present with complex posttraumatic conditions and associated comorbidities (Marotta-Walters, Jain, DiNardo, Kaur, & Kaligounder, 2018). With EMDR mHealth applications, the EMDR-trained clinicians can attach headphones to a mobile phone device and then use the application to administer bilateral tones to the client. In alternative versions, the therapist will play the application on a computer, providing the client with both visual and auditory bilateral stimulation (Lee & Cuijpers, 2013).

As individuals adapt to survive during the COVID-19 global pandemic, the potential dangers associated with this kind of technology cannot be disregarded. There are currently no federal or state agencies overseeing the confidentiality of data collected by mHealth applications, which are available in mobile application stores. The Federal Communications Commission (FCC), the Food and Drug Administration (FDA), and the Office of Civil Rights can only regulate mHealth applications when the applications interact or exchange personally identifiable data, according to the Health Insurance Portability and Accountability Act (HIPAA) (Marotta-Walters et al., 2018). Marotta-Walters et al. (2018) caution that easy accessibility to unregulated mHealth applications for the treatment of severe mental health issues such as complex trauma poses a number of serious risks, including a lack of HIPAA-compliant data privacy and security. These applications also have potential to cause psychological harm to clients if used improperly, including triggering dissociation and emotional dysregulation. EMDR clinicians are trained to work with clients' associated memories and to optimize potential transformative changes (known as interweaves) to the targeted memory. Without therapeutic guidance, it is possible that many individuals would be unable to fulfill this component of treatment (Hofmann & Barlow, 2014; Wampold, 2015). The originator of EMDR, Francine Shapiro (2018), has warned that it is impossible for individuals to engage in intense, complex personal therapy without an EMDR-trained therapist's assistance. Shapiro (2018) does not recommend that clients be taught the self-directed use of eye movements, as without the guidance of a trained EMDR therapist, uncovering how target memories, somatic disturbances, and emotions are linked will not be feasible.

In January 2020, the EMDR International Association's "Report of the Virtual Training and Therapy Task Group" was released, with the intention of providing clearer direction concerning best Virtual EMDR (VEMDR) practices. In this report, references to virtual delivery of EMDR therapy pertain exclusively to EMDR therapy that is administered by an EMDR-trained clinician online via HIPAA-compliant telecommunications that have a Business Associate Agreement (BAA). References to VEMDR in the report do not concern companies, websites, or services that offer EMDR self-therapy without live guidance from an EMDR-trained clinician. Mirroring the concerns expressed by Marotta-Walters et al. (2018), self-administration of EMDR therapy is strictly forbidden in the policies outlined in this report. Additionally, this task group highlighted the necessity for EMDR-trained clinicians to complete a tele-mental health certification in order to maintain a safe standard of online practice, prior to providing VEMDR. The task group further recommended that EMDR clinicians stay abreast of the rapidly changing technologies and guidelines in order to adequately maintain safety and security within their practice. Along with these technology guidelines, the task group recommended that EMDR clinicians providing virtual treatment must demonstrate online attunement, ethical integrity, and fidelity to the EMDR therapy model. While EMDR-trained clinicians are guided to be attentive to the client's safety and comfort level during reprocessing, the report warned that VEMDR presents special risk for misattunement because of limited eye contact, limited visual cues (noticing motor activity), and the forfeiture of the in-person connection.

These risks are evident across all modalities, including TF-CBT, SP, and SE. Both SP and SE are focused strongly on attunement, resonance, and connection which can prove to be helpful in anchoring clients during the social isolation caused by COVID-19. However, a clinician can only observe the face and upper bilateral motor activity during these remote sessions, which deprives the clinician of information related to upper motor activity and associated affect regulation cues. This makes it especially critical for clinicians to build strong attunement and communication skills to ensure optimal connection with the client during telepsychotherapy, while recognizing that this process is rife with challenges, given unavoidable technical glitches and/or unclear processing (O'Shea Brown 2021). This is especially true for clients suffering from complex trauma, as technological malfunctions, such as frozen screen, can appear eerily similar to the "Still Face Experiment." The "Still Face Experiment" was conducted by placing an infant face to face with their non-responsive, expressionless mother following 3 min of free interaction (Tronick, Als, Adamson, Wise, & Brazelton, 1978; Tronick & Gold, 2020). After repeated attempts to engage their mother, the infant typically withdraws and orients their face and body away from the mother with a withdrawn, hopeless facial expression. When connectivity issues occur, the clinician may miss a client's cues and inadvertently replicate this experience in emotionally vulnerable clients, potentially impacting the client-clinician dyad and causing undue stress and potential retraumatization.

To counteract this risk, Watson-Wong (2013) has advised that prior to beginning reprocessing, clinicians should build an alliance with a client's adult ego state to enable helpful communication and evaluate missed or confusing cues and clues during processing. Clinicians should apply their transferable skills of building strong attunement and empathic listening, to help clients stay engaged and connected during telepsychotherapy. Empathic listening and understanding occurs when a clinician paraphrases or summarizes a client's comments to foster connection and trust. In addition to ensuring that the client feels heard and understood, this technique has a secondary gain of allowing the client the opportunity to correct the clinician if they have in some way misinterpreted their insights. Self-determination and the therapeutic alliance have repeatedly been shown to greatly enhance the efficacy of psychotherapy treatment across all modalities (Davidson, 2006; Marsh, Angell, Andrews, & Curry, 2012; Stanhope, Barrenger, Salzer, & Marcus, 2013). Therefore, guiding the client to be more involved in the treatment process and clinical decision-making will ultimately enhance the clinical outcome by promoting a sense of agency and empowerment, regardless of the chosen modality. This is especially applicable to clinicians who are adapting their therapeutic practice in the wake of COVID-19.

Ultimately if this trust is fostered and maintained over the course of the clinical relationship, it will provide a much-needed place of safety for the survivor to continue their healing process, even in spite of the challenges of conducting therapy remotely.

Summary

Research has consistently shown that the treatment of complex trauma should be phase-oriented, multimodal, and skill-focused, with a core emphasis on symptom relief and functional improvement (Briere & Scott, 2006; Courtois et al., 2009; van der Kolk, 2015).

Within this holistic, integrative framework, there is an appreciation of the mind-body connection. Complex trauma treatment has evolved into a more integrative, body-oriented approach through modalities such as Eye Movement Desensitization and Reprocessing (Shapiro, 1989), Sensorimotor Psychotherapy (Ogden, Minton, et al. 2006), and Somatic Experiencing (Levine, 1997). These modalities offer interventions that can be used autonomously by clients to enhance self-empowered healing of the mind and body. Self-determination and the therapeutic alliance have repeatedly been shown to greatly enhance the efficacy of psychotherapy treatment across all modalities (Davidson, 2006; Marsh et al., 2012; Stanhope et al., 2013). Therefore, guiding the client to be more involved in the treatment process and clinical decision-making will ultimately enhance the clinical outcome by promoting a sense of agency and empowerment, regardless of the chosen modality.

Questions and Activities for Discussion and Further Reflection

1. Class will be divided into groups, and each group will work together to create a 5-minute presentation providing a synopsis of one of the following topics: TF-CBT, EMDR, Sensorimotor Psychotherapy, Somatic Experiencing, and telepsychotherapy.
2. Assignment: Choose one modality to write about by exploring its inception, its positive and negative aspects, and the research on its efficacy.
3. Class Discussion Prompt: Reflect on the modalities you have been reading about. Discuss the pros and cons of each.
4. Have an open discussion on whether you would be interested in advancing your knowledge in a particular modality through training or certification. If yes, what makes this intervention more attractive to you than the others?

References

Ahmad, A., Larsson, B., & Sundelin-Wahlsten, V. (2007). EMDR treatment for children with PTSD: Results of a randomized controlled trial. *Nordic Journal of Psychiatry, 61*, 349–354.

American Psychiatric Association. (2013). *Diagnostic and statistical manual of mental disorders* (5th ed.). Washington, DC: American Psychiatric Publishing.

Bisson, J. I. (2009). The neurobiology of posttraumatic stress disorder. *Psychiatry, 8*(8), 288–289.

Bowlby, J. (1989). The role of attachment in personality development and psychopathology. In S. I. Greenspan & G. H. Pollack (Eds.), *The course of life: Vol. 1. Infancy* (pp. 119–136). Madison, WI: International Universities Press.

Briere, J., & Scott, C. (2006). *Principles of trauma therapy: A guide to symptoms, evaluation, and treatment*. London, UK: Sage.

Brom, D., Stokar, Y., Lawi, C., Nuriel-Porat, V., Ziv, Y., Lerner, K., & Ross, G. (2017). Somatic experiencing for posttraumatic stress disorder: A randomized controlled outcome study. *Journal of Traumatic Stress, 30*(3), 304–312. https://doi.org/10.1002/jts.22189

Chen, R., Gillespie, A., Zhao, Y., Xi, Y., Ren, Y., & McLean, L. (2018). The efficacy of eye movement desensitization and reprocessing in children and adults who have experienced complex childhood trauma: A systematic review of randomized controlled trials. *Frontiers in Psychology, 9*, 534. https://doi.org/10.3389/fpsyg.2018.00534

Cohen, J. A., Deblinger, E., Mannarino, A. P., & Steer, R. (2004). A multisite, randomized controlled trial for children with sexual abuse related PTSD symptoms. *Journal of the American Academy of Child and Adolescent Psychiatry, 43*, 393–402. https://doi.org/10.1097/01.chi.0000111364.94169.f9

Cohen, J. A., Mannarino, A. P., & Deblinger, E. (2006). *Treating trauma and traumatic grief in children and adolescents*. New York, NY: Guilford Press.

Cohen, J. A., Mannarino, A. P., & Knudsen, K. (2005). Treating sexually abused children: One year follow-up of a randomized controlled trial. *Child Abuse and Neglect, 29*, 135–145. https://doi.org/10.1016/jchiabu.2004.12.005

Courtois, C. A., Ford, J. D., & Cloitre, M. (2009). Best practices in psychotherapy for adults. In C. A. Courtois & J. D. Ford (Eds.), *Treating complex traumatic stress disorders: An evidence-based guide* (pp. 82–103). New York, NY: Guilford Press.

Davidson, L. (2006). The top ten concerns about recovery encountered in mental health system transformation. Psychiatric Services. 2006;57:640–645. doi: https://doi.org/10.1176/appi.ps.57.5.640.

Deblinger, E., Mannarino, A. P., Cohen, J. A., & Steer, R. (2006). A follow-up study of a multisite randomized controlled trial for children with sexual abuse related PTSD symptoms. *Journal of the American Academy of Child and Adolescent Psychiatry, 45*, 1474–1484. https://doi.org/10.1097/01.chi.0000240839.56114.bb

Drisko, J., & Grady, M. (2019). *Evidence-based practice in clinical social work*. Switzerland: Springer.

Fisher, J. (2001). *Modified EMDR resource development & installation protocol*. Presentation at the trauma Center, Boston, MA.

Fisher, J. (2002). *Adapting EMDR techniques in the treatment of dysregulated or dissociative patients*. Paper presented at the International Society for the Study of Dissociation Annual Meeting, San Antonio, Texas November 12, 2000.

Fisher, J. (2019). Sensorimotor psychotherapy in the treatment of trauma. *Practice Innovations, 4*(3), 156–165. https://doi.org/10.1037/pri0000096

Ford, J., Courtois, C. A., Steele, K., van der Hart, O., & Nijenhuis, E. R. S. (2005). Treatment of complex posttraumatic self-dysregulation. *Journal of Traumatic Stress, 18*, 437–447.

Forgash, C., & Copeley, M. (2008). *Healing the heart of trauma and dissociation with EMDR and ego state therapy*, New York, Springer.

Forte, G., Favieri, F., Tambelli, R., & Casagrande, M. (2020). COVID-19 pandemic in the Italian population: Validation of a post-traumatic stress disorder questionnaire and prevalence of

PTSD symptomatology. *International Journal of Environmental Research and Public Health, 17*(11), 4151. https://doi.org/10.3390/ijerph17114151

Gene-Cos, N., Fisher, J., Ogden, P., & Cantrell, A. (2016). Sensorimotor group therapy in the treatment of complex PTSD. *Annals of Psychiatry and Mental Health, 4*, 1080.

Harvey, A. G., Bryant, R. A., & Tarrier, N. (2003). Cognitive behaviour therapy for posttraumatic stress disorder. *Clinical Psychology Review, 23*, 501–522. https://doi.org/10.1016/S0272-7258(03)00035-7

Herman, J. L. (1992). *Trauma and recovery: The aftermath of violence*. New York, NY: Basic Books.

Hilty, D. M., Ferrer, D. C., Parish, M. B., Johnston, B., Callahan, E. J., & Yellowless, P. M. (2013). The effectiveness of telemental health: A 2013 review. *Telemedicine and e-Health, 19*(6), 444–454.

Hofmann, S. G., & Barlow, D. H. (2014). Evidence-based psychological interventions and the common factors approach: The beginnings of a rapprochement. *Psychotherapy, 51*(4), 510–513. https://doi.org/10.1037/a0037045

Jensen, T. K., Holt, T., Ormhaug, S. M., Egeland, K., Granly, L., Hoaas, L. C., & Wentzel-Larsen, T. (2014). A randomized effectiveness study comparing trauma-focused cognitive behavioral therapy with therapy as usual for youth. *Journal of Clinical Child and Adolescent Psychology, 43*(3), 356–369. https://doi.org/10.1080/15374416.2013.822307

Kang, L., Ma, S., Chen, M., Yang, J., Wang, Y., Li, R., … Liu, Z. (2020). Impact on mental health and perceptions of psychological care among medical and nursing staff in Wuhan during the 2019 novel coronavirus disease outbreak: A cross-sectional study. *Brain, Behavior, and Immunity*. https://doi.org/10.1016/j.bbi.2020.03.028

Korn, D. L. (2009). EMDR and the treatment of complex PTSD: A review. *Journal of EMDR Practice and Research, 3*(4), 264–278. https://doi.org/10.1891/1933-3196.3.4.264

Korn, D. L., & Leeds, A. M. (2002). Preliminary evidence of efficacy for EMDR resource development and installation in the stabilization phase of treatment of complex posttraumatic stress disorder. *Journal of Clinical Psychology, 58*(12), 1465–1487. https://doi.org/10.1002/jclp.10099

Kramer, G. M., Shore, J. H., Mishkind, M. C., Friedl, K. E., Poropatich, R. K., & Gahm, G. A. (2012). A standard telemental health evaluation model: The time is now. *Telemedicine and e-Health, 18*(4), 309–313.

Langarizadeh, M., Tabatabaei, M. S., Tavakol, K., Naghipour, M., Rostami, A., & Moghbeli, F. (2017). Telemental health care, an effective alternative to conventional mental care: A systematic review. *Acta Informatic Medica, 25*(4), 240.

Langmuir, J., Kirsh, S., & Classen, C. (2012). A pilot study of body-oriented group psychotherapy: Adapting sensorimotor psychotherapy for the group treatment of trauma. *Psychological Trauma: Theory, Research, Practice, and Policy, 4*, 145–151. https://doi.org/10.1037/a0025588

Lanius, R. A., Vermetten, E., Loewenstein, R. J., Brand, B., Schmahl, C., Bremner, J., & Speigel, D. (2010, June). Emotion modulation in PTSD: Clinical and neurobiological evidence for a dissociative subtype. *American Journal of Psychiatry, 167*(6), 640–647. https://doi.org/10.1176/appi.ajp.209.09081168 National Center for PTSD (2011, February).

Lee, C. W., & Cuijpers, P. (2013). A meta-analysis of the contribution of eye movements in processing emotional memories. *Journal of Behavior Therapy and Experimental Psychiatry, 44*(2), 231–239. https://doi.org/10.1016/j.jbtep.2012.11.001

Leeds, A. M. (1995). *EMDR case formulation symposium*. Paper presented at the annual meeting of the International EMDR Association, Santa Monica.

Leeds, A. M., & Shapiro, F. (2000). EMDR ad Resource Installation: Principles and procedures for enhancing current functioning and resolving traumatic experiences. In J. Carlson & L. Sperry (Eds.), *Brief therapy strategies with individuals and couples* (pp. 469–534). Phoenix, AZ: Zeig, Tucker, Theisen, Inc.

Levine, P. (1997). *Waking the Tiger: Healing trauma*. Berkeley, CA: North Atlantic Books.

Levine, P. A. (1977). *Accumulated stress, reserve capacity and disease*. Ann Arbor, MI: University of California. Berkeley.

Levine, P. A. (2010). *In an unspoken voice: How the body releases trauma and restores goodness.* Berkeley, CA: North Atlantic Books.
Marcus, S., Marquis, P., & Sakai, C. (2004). Three- and 6-month follow-up of EMDR treatment of PTSD in an HMO setting. *International Journal of Stress Management, 11*(3), 195–208. https://doi.org/10.1037/1072-5245.11.3.195
Marotta-Walters, S. A., Jain, K., DiNardo, J., Kaur, P., & Kaligounder, S. (2018). A review of mobile applications for facilitating EMDR treatment of complex trauma and its comorbidities. *Journal of EMDR Practice and Research, 12*(1). https://doi.org/10.1891/1933-3196.12.1.2
Marsh, J. C., Angell, B., Andrews, C. M., & Curry, A. (2012). Client-provider relationship and treatment outcome: A systematic review of substance abuse, child welfare, and mental health services research. *Journal of the Society for Social Work and Research, 3*, 233–267. https://doi.org/10.5243/jsswr.2012.15
Masero, M. (2017). The wisdom of the body and couple therapy – A sensorimotor psychotherapy perspective: An interview with Pat Ogden. *The Australian and New Zealand Journal of Family Therapy, 38*(4), 657–668. https://doi.org/10.1002/anzf.1267
O'Shea Brown, G. (2020). Internal family systems informed eye movement desensitization and reprocessing: An integrative technique for treatment of complex posttraumatic stress disorder. *International Body Psychotherapy Journal, 19*(2), 112–122.
O'Shea Brown, G. (2021). Reflections on providing virtual eye movement desensitization and reprocessing therapy in the wake of COVID-19: Survival through adaptation. In C. Tosone (Ed.), *Shared trauma, Shared resilience during a pandemic: Social work in the time of COVID-19*. Cham, Switzerland: Springer.
Ogden, P., & Fisher, J. (2006). A sensorimotor approach to the treatment of trauma and dissociation. *Psychiatric Clinics of North America, 29*(1), 263–279. xi–xii.
Ogden, P., Minton, K., & Pain, C. (2006). *Trauma and the body: A sensorimotor approach to psychotherapy*. New York, NY: Norton.
Ogden, P., Pain, C., & Fisher, J. (2006). A sensorimotor approach to the treatment of trauma and dissociation. *Psychiatric Clinics of North America, 29*, 263–279.
Pappa, S., Ntella, V., Giannakas, T., Giannakoulis, V. G., Papoutsi, E., & Katsaounou, P. (2020). Prevalence of depression, anxiety, and insomnia among healthcare workers during the COVID-19 pandemic: A systematic review and meta-analysis. *Brain, Behavior, and Immunity.* https://doi.org/10.1016/j.bbi.2020.05.026
Parker, C., Doctor, R. M., & Selvam, R. (2008). Somatic therapy treatment effects with tsunami survivors. *Traumatology, 14*, 103–109. https://doi.org/10.1177/1534765608319080
Payne, P., Levine, P. A., & Crane-Godreau, M. A. (2015). Somatic experiencing: Using interoception and proprioception as core elements of trauma therapy. *Frontiers in Psychology, 6*, 93. https://doi.org/10.3389/fpsyg.2015.00093
Schore, A. (2003). *Affect regulation and the repair of the self.* New York, NY: Norton.
Shapiro, F. (1989). Efficacy of the eye movement desensitization procedure in the treatment of traumatic memories. *Journal of Traumatic Stress, 2*, 199–223. https://doi.org/10.1002/jts.2490020207
Shapiro, F. (1991). Eye movement desensitization and reprocessing: From EMD to EMDR/R – a new treatment model for anxiety and related traumata. *The Behavior Therapist, 14*(5), 133–135.
Shapiro, F. (1995). *Eye movement desensitization and reprocessing, basic principles, protocols and procedures*. New York, NY: Guilford Press.
Shapiro, F. (2001). *Eye movement desensitization and reprocessing: Basic principles, protocols, and procedures* (2nd ed.). New York, NY: Guilford Press.
Shapiro, F. (2007). EMDR, adaptive information processing, and case conceptualization. *Journal of EMDR Practice and Research, 1*(2), 68–87. https://doi.org/10.1891/1933-3196.1.2.68
Shapiro, F. (2018). *Eye Movement Desensitization and Reprocessing (EMDR) therapy: Basic principles protocols, and procedures* (3rd ed., pp. 243–244). New York, NY: Guilford Press.
Shigemura, J., Ursano, R. J., Morganstein, J. C., Kurosawa, M., & Benedek, D. M. (2020). Public responses to the novel 2019 coronavirus (2019 – nCoV): Mental health consequences and target populations. *Psychiatry and Clinical Neurosciences.* [Epub ahead of print]

Siegel, D. (1999). *The developing mind: Toward a neurobiology of interpersonal experience*. New York, NY: Guilford Press.
Stanhope, V., Barrenger, S. L., Salzer, M. S., & Marcus, S. C. (2013). Examining the relationship between choice, therapeutic alliance and outcomes in mental health services. *Journal of personalized medicine, 3*(3), 191–202. https://doi.org/10.3390/jpm3030191
Stickgold, R. (2002). EMDR: A putative neurobiological mechanism of action. *Journal of Clinical Psychology, 58*(1), 61–75. https://doi.org/10.1002/jclp.1129
Tan, B. Y. Q., Chew, N. W. S., Lee, G. K. H., Jing, M., Goh, Y., Yeo, L. L. L., … Sharma, V. K. (2020). Psychological Impact of the COVID-19 Pandemic on 2 9 Health Care Workers in Singapore. *Annals of Internal Medicine*. https://doi.org/10.7326/M20-1083
Tronick, E., Als, H., Adamson, L., Wise, S., & Brazelton, T. B. (1978). Infants' response to entrapment between contradictory messages in face-to-face interaction. *Journal of the American Academy of Child and Adolescent Psychiatry, 17*, 1–13.
Tronick, E., & Gold, C. (2020). *The power of discord: Why ups and downs of relationships are the secret to building intimacy, resilience, and trust*. New York, NY: Hachette Book Club.
Twombly, J. H., & Schwartz, R. C. (2008). The integration of the internal family systems model and EMDR. In C. Forgash & M. Copeley (Eds.), *Healing the heart of trauma and dissociation with EMDR and ego state therapy* (pp. 295–311). New York, NY: Springer Publishing Co..
van der Kolk, B. A. (2015). *The body keeps the score: Brain, mind and body in the healing of trauma*. New York, NY: Viking Press.
van der Kolk, B. A., McFarlane, A., & Weisaeth, L. (1996). *Traumatic stress*. New York, NY: Guilford Press.
Wampold, B. E. (2015). How important are the common factors in psychotherapy? An update. *World Psychiatry, 14*(3), 270–277. https://doi.org/10.1002/wps.20238
Watson-Wong, J. (2013, September). *Poster titled, EMDR internet therapy, presented at the 18th EMDR International Association Conference*. Austin, TX.
Wilson, S. A., Becker, L. A., & Tinker, R. H. (1997). Fifteen-month follow-up of eye movement desensitization and reprocessing (EMDR) treatment for posttraumatic stress disorder and psychological trauma. *Journal of Consulting and Clinical Psychology, 65*(6), 1047–1056.
Winblad, N. E., Changaris, M., & Stein, P. K. (2018). Effect of somatic experiencing resiliency-based trauma treatment training on quality of life and psychological health as potential markers of resilience in treating professionals. *Frontiers Neuroscience*. https://doi.org/10.3389/fnins.2018.00070
World Health Organization [WHO]. (2013). *Guidelines for the management of conditions specifically related to stress*. Geneva, Switzerland: WHO.
Zandifar, A., & Badrfam, R. (2020). Iranian mental health during the COVID-19 epidemic. *Asian Journal of Psychiatry, 51*, 101990.

Chapter 9
Ego State Work and Connecting with the Inner Child

As the treatment of complex trauma deepens, it is inevitable that by peeling back the layers of self-discovery, you will encounter the inner child. Carl Jung is credited with coining the term "inner child." Jung (1940/1958) proclaimed that within every adult exists an eternal child that is perpetually in a state of becoming more and requires nurturing through unceasing care, attention, and education. The inner child is the part of us that is vulnerable, creative, playful, expressive, and in need of tenderness. Jung (1940/1958) explained that the divine child archetype resides within all of us and contended that by accessing the inner child, we can pave the way for deeper healing, in addition to more profound behavioral and emotional change.

Figure 9.1 is a photo of a sculpture created by Ukrainian artist Alexander Milov, entitled "Love," which was first exhibited at Burning Man Festival in 2015. This sculpture portrays two adults sitting back to back, despondent and resentful after a disagreement. At times of great personal distress, the reclusive and independent nature of the adult self can create a barrier to connection. In this sculpture, the outer expression of despondency is juxtaposed with the depiction of the inner child of each figure, reaching outward and seeking comfort and clemency through connection with the other, undeterred by pride or resentment.

There are times in the therapeutic dyad when a client may outwardly respond with hostility, avoidance, or uncertainty, and it is during these pivotal moments that a compassionate and gentle approach is most needed (O'Shea Brown, 2020). A multi-consciousness approach to clinical treatment enables the trauma survivor to hear from the various parts of their own consciousness through a compassionate lens, which can ultimately pave the way for negotiation, clarity, and inner harmony. Thoughtful application of ego-state-informed language can facilitate compassionate, nonjudgmental witnessing of the parts that are coming to voice so that they can be heard and even unburdened of their fears. This chapter will begin by exploring the relationship between trauma and the multiplicity of the mind, illustrated through a clinical vignette. Subsequently, an overview of the theoretical underpinning and application of the Internal Family Systems Model will be provided.

G. O'Shea Brown, *Healing Complex Posttraumatic Stress Disorder*, Essential Clinical Social Work Series, https://doi.org/10.1007/978-3-030-61416-4_9

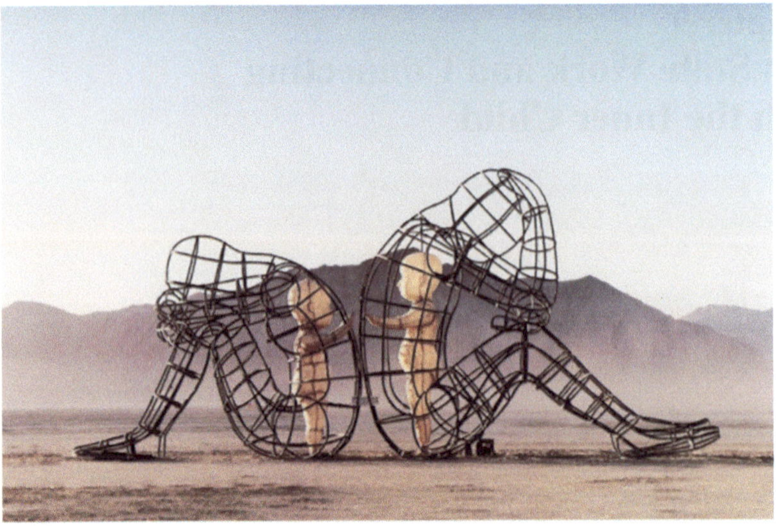

Fig. 9.1 A sculpture entitled "Love" by © Alexander Milov exhibited at Burning Man Festival in 2015. All Rights Reserved. Photograph by Gerome Viavant. (Published with kind permission of artist and photographer. Photograph licensed under the terms of the Creative Commons Attribution License (https://creativecommons.org/licenses/by/4.0/))

Trauma and the Multiplicity of the Mind

Chronic traumatization, especially in the formative years, leaves a legacy that often results in trauma survivors presenting with a fragmented sense of self (Janet, 1889). Dissociative splitting is a natural part of trauma: it allows the individual to survive in a precarious environment through the use of cognitive dissonance (Siegel, 1999; van Der Hart, Nijenhuis, Steele, & Brown, 2004). Trauma-related splitting and compartmentalization enable trauma survivors to distance from certain undesirable parts of the self by creating a dissociative wall, which can provide relief from the painful remnants of trauma. However, dissociative splitting can lead to the application of selective attention, and, thus, internal conflicts can be left unresolved and implicit memories suppressed (van der Hart, Nijenhuis, & Steele, 2006). The fragmented self enables the trauma survivor to validate their survival rather than ruminate on their perceived failure or deficit.

The multiplicity of the mind has been explored by various therapeutic modalities that work with ego states or "parts," for instance, Ego State Therapy (Watkins and Watkins, 1997), Gestalt Therapy (Perls, 1973), and Internal Family Systems (IFS) therapy (Schwartz, 1995). The ultimate goal of ego state work is to transform the internal dialogue between the parts of the self from disjointed chaos to a smooth, harmonic symphony. Parts-type therapy is based on the concept that our personality is composed of various personality parts which are aspects of the subconscious, each with their own respective jobs or functions within the inner mind. Exploring parts helps clients to resolve internal conflicts by drawing upon their own internal knowledge and capabilities. Additionally, for many trauma survivors, therapy represents a stable, predictable, reliable, and trustworthy foundation that instantiates a sense of trust and connection (O'Shea Brown, 2021).

Fraser's Dissociative Table Technique (1991) facilitates access to ego states and offers additional strategies to apply family therapy interventions to these fragmented parts of self to foster internal healing. This technique enables clients to recognize internal ego states and to structure and control internal communication. Clients are instructed to identify alliances and conflicts among the various parts of self. By exploring and compassionately connecting with different facets of their own character, clients can begin to work through internal conflicts and even work with certain disowned or undesirable parts.

Case Study

This following composite case study demonstrates Eduardo[1], a 32-year-old Latinx male with a history of childhood trauma, being guided through Fraser's Dissociative Table Technique. Eduardo presented to therapy struggling with symptoms of shame and dissociation due to his past history of relational trauma and emotional abuse. Despite his gregarious demeanor, he reports that he often feels "numb" and disconnected from those around him. He reports frequent prolonged exposure to domestic disputes in his formative years. After being guided through a relaxation exercise, Eduardo is guided toward meeting with his "parts," as shown in the excerpt below. Through this technique, he is able to identify various parts of self, and subsequently a language can be developed to pave the way toward conflict resolution and internal harmony.

Clinician: We need to find a way to communicate with all the various parts of you. Everyone has "parts" or facets of self. These parts vie for airtime and contribute to the conflicting feelings and chronic struggles that you may have. You have heard the language, "One part of me feels sad and another part feels mad" or "On one hand I want this, but on the other hand I want that." It will be helpful to identify these various factions of yourself to help us to resolve the issues that you wish to resolve. Are you willing to give this a try?

Eduardo: (nods)

Clinician: Now I would like you to leave your calm state and imagine a room with a table in it. This room is a pleasant room where no harm can come to you. The table in this room is a special table. It can be as big or as small as you need, with just the right number of chairs. When you have the image of this table, let me know by nodding.

Eduardo: (nods)

[1] A pseudonym has been used to preserve confidentiality.

Clinician: Now I want you to imagine walking into this room and taking your place at the table. When you are settled in, I want you to let me know by nodding.

Eduardo: (nods)

Clinician: Now I want you to invite all of the various aspects or parts of yourself to come into this room and take their places at the table. Watch them as they come in one by one. If they cannot come in, perhaps they can stay on the side-lines or in an adjoining room. When they are all there, I want you to let me know by nodding.

Eduardo: (nods)

Clinician: Who and what do you see?

Eduardo: I am sitting at the top of the table. It is a rectangular table. There is a glass partition dividing the room. On the other side, there is a pacing detective. He looks pensive, and highly anxious. I am sitting at the table. Next to me, there is a younger version of me. He looks angry and annoyed. He is in his early teens, I think 14. He is slouched over and clenching his jaw and his fists. Next to him is a worn-out, depleted, young professional me. I think it's me after graduate school at about 22 years old. He has no energy and feels exhausted. There's also a very little me, he is about 6 years old and he plays on the floor with his toys, oblivious to all of us. On the other side of me there is the passionate one; this is the part of me that comes out when I am in creative flow. This part is energized, focused, and powerful. It is a healing voice, sending me messages of love and encouragement.

Clinician: Good Job, Eduardo. Take a few breaths and notice what you observe. Notice any dialogue occurring…or any conflicts or alliances between the parts.

Eduardo: There is a general fear toward the teenager. He makes the other parts feel uncomfortable because of his rage. The passionate one is engaging the little boy and the others seem bewildered as to why they are there.

Clinician: Okay, notice what you are experiencing and witnessing.

Eduardo: Yes, it feels like a lot right now, but I would like to get to know these parts over time.

Clinician: All parts are welcome and all parts are valuable.

As we get to know them more, we will learn their role, purpose, and function. We will also learn about conflicts and alliances.

When we hear from these parts we may learn about their core beliefs and fears. If you want to stay and explore more we can; however, if you have experienced enough for today you can thank the parts for showing up, let them know you will continue to get to know them, and say goodbye in your own special way.

Then slowly get up, walk toward the door, twist the knob and open your eyes as you reenter this room.

Fraser's Dissociative Table Technique (1991) allows access to ego states and offers additional strategies to work with them. However, it is important to note that this is not a therapy modality in itself, but rather a strategy that can be used in conjunction with the clinical approach of the clinician knowledgeable in ego states. This adaptation of Fraser's Dissociative Table Technique has been used only as a means to introduce you to the multiplicity of the mind, as if it were a mosaic connected but fragmented (it is generally not applied to the later discussed IFS model). A parts-type approach offers a delicate way to deepen trauma work. From here a clinician can apply their family therapy skills to resolve internal conflicts and power imbalances and hear from all parts equally.

Survivors of childhood abuse perpetrated by a parent often feel as though they are walking on a tight rope, attempting to strike a delicate balance between avoidance of further pain and a desire to resolve trauma. For some survivors, complete estrangement from the family abuser evokes feelings of guilt; however, getting too close increases the risk of retraumatization. A multi-consciousness approach to clinical treatment enables the trauma survivor to hear from the various parts through a compassionate lens, which can ultimately pave the way for negotiation, clarity, and inner harmony. This subsequent section will explore the theoretical underpinning and application of the Internal Family Systems Model. The overview of this modality does not supplement the required training and certification to use the modality (information on which is listed in the Appendix).

The Internal Family Systems Model

In 1995, Richard Schwartz, PhD, pioneered the Internal Family Systems (IFS) Model, which applies family systems theory to the integration of sub-personalities or parts of self in order to access an internal self-leadership quality. The IFS model represents a synthesis of two already-existing paradigms: systems thinking and the multiplicity of the mind. However, what makes IFS unique among modalities working with ego states is the belief that everyone has a self-leadership quality which, when accessed, allows for a relationship with all parts, preventing the patient from being hijacked by a renegade aspect of the self. The IFS model proposes the universal presence of an untarnished self within everyone; this self, referred to as "self-energy," encompasses qualities of calmness, curiosity, compassion, confidence, courage, clarity, connectedness, and creativity (Schwartz, 2001; Schwartz & Sweezy, 2020). IFS posits that harnessing self-leadership leads to inherent healing and self-wisdom. Once established, the self develops a relationship with each ego state so it can help lead them in efforts to heal the exiled or traumatized inner child.

The IFS model posits that in addition to the self, there is an ecology of relatively discrete, autonomous parts or ego states that each contain a unique quality and perform a valuable role. Each part has developed during the individual's life for a specific reason and purpose. Every part has positive intentions for the person, even if actions at times are perceived as resistant, dysfunctional, or maladaptive. "Managers" are parts that manage an individual's interactions within their external environment in order to protect them from pain or retraumatization. In traditional psychodynamic therapy, the manager would be characterized as the individual's defense mechanisms. Similar to parentified children, these manager parts protect more vulnerable parts in the system by being orderly, disciplined, and at times controlling (Twombly & Schwartz, 2008). In the table exercise, the manager is the pacing detective who looks pensive and highly anxious. His role is to be alert for any event that might cause psychic harm. During such times, his anxiety takes center stage. "Exiles" are disowned parts that are in active pain, shame, or fear. They are the traumatized parts that need healing. In the exercise, the exile is the little child part of about 6 years old who is playing on the floor with his toys, oblivious to all—in other words, dissociated. This is also the inner child embedded in the mesh sculptures (Fig. 9.1).

"Firefighters" are parts that emerge when managers become overwhelmed or exiles are exposed. The primary role of firefighters is to divert or suppress pain, which is usually achieved through ritualistic, compulsive comfort-seeking behavior or risky action urges. Therefore, firefighters tend to be dominant in people who live with addiction (Schwartz, 2001). In the table exercise, this is the 14-year-old part who is clenching his jaw and fists, ready for a fight to divert attention to protect the hurt child. It is also the passionate one, whose creative energetic flow powerfully transcends the traumatized child—as though saying, "Look at me! Leave the child alone."

In IFS, healing occurs in a series of methodical steps. The initial phase of the IFS treatment process is to differentiate or "unblend" parts from the self. When parts become "blended" with the self, they may eclipse the self and take over. No work can be done. The major question used to assess whether the self is leading is to ask the client, "How do you feel toward the part?" This helps to create a boundary between the self and a part, a differentiation from which a relationship can begin.

After accessing the self and building its ability to lead, the self begins the process of compassionately "witnessing" each of the parts. The various parts are asked if they have any objections to the work. Once permission is earned and agreement is established, the process of compassionate "witnessing" can occur. The clinician may guide compassionate witnessing by asking, "What does the part fear will happen if it doesn't do its job?" The fears held by each part propel it to rigidly fulfill its function. Other questions asked during compassionate witnessing may include: "What does the part have to say? What is their secret history? What do they protect?" These parts control emotions and sensations. They control the outside world and how the person looks and performs. They make sure the person does not get hurt. Each part needs to be witnessed and honored for their role, so that their value is known and recognized. They will not step aside or leave their roles until the self befriends and understands them. The most important mission of the self is to become curious and calm in order to engage in meaningful dialogue and connect with each part. Our job is to heal the parts from their burdens and appreciate what they protect.

Once the parts feel known, respected, and understood, they may agree to step aside, and from here the exile work can begin. The exiles carry the shame, memories, sensations, and emotions of the traumatic events stuck in the past, deep down in the pit. Exiles thus require nurturing through unceasing care, attention, and education. The exile is the part of us that is vulnerable, creative, playful, expressive, and in need of tenderness. They are also the most loving and spontaneous, precious part. The exile, the child in the table exercise above, needs the self to really get what happened at the traumatic moment when they were hurt: to understand how bad it was, to absorb the magnitude of what the child endured. This serves the function of *witnessing*. The clinician can ask questions to guide the client in addressing the exile or child. For example, "Can you ask the child if they want to show you what happened back then? What is the child concerned would happen if it showed you that memory? Is there anything else the child wants to show you?" In order to heal, the trauma not only needs to be witnessed, but it must also be retrieved from the past. "Retrieval" is the process by which the self takes a part out of the past and into the present. The clinician may ask, "Can you ask that part to go into the scene and be with that young child in the way they needed to be with at that time?"

Next, the process of "unburdening" begins. The burdens that parts carry, rather than the parts themselves, cause problems in the internal system. Therefore, parts must be unburdened for deep healing to occur, and parts must be guided to process and release emotions. The exile is asked if there are extreme thoughts or feelings they took on from the painful past experience. "Is there anything in or around the child's body that they are carrying? Something that isn't appropriate for the child to carry anymore?" Many times, this can be a heaviness, guilt, or sense of shame. "Can you ask the child to let go of that? Is there anything you can do to help the child let go of that burden? Sometimes parts release burdens by burning them, releasing them into the wind, burying them, or releasing them to the water, but you can get a sense for yourself how the child wishes to release the burden. After the burden has been released, the clinician can enquire compassionately: "How does that part feel now?"

Finally, in the "invitation" phase, the client asks the part to invite back any resources or qualities that would be helpful for them in the future. Integration involves checking in with the part to see what it might want or need from the self in the days to come. "Please check inside to see if there is anything else that needs to happen (particularly with parts that agreed to step back). Thank those parts for stepping back. Do they want another role?"

IFS provides an essential language to access and understand the parts of the self, in addition to working through any unresolved internal conflicts. The IFS-trained clinician works as an ally alongside the client's self, which eventually becomes the compassionate therapist and leader of the family system. The IFS model creates a language for trauma survivors to affirm and unburden their parts, allowing their self to lead the way. The gentle, affirmative language of IFS, combined with its focused strategies, can help the client to go deeper so that profound healing can occur (Schwartz, 2001).

Case Study

The following case study is a composite case that contains elements and techniques derived from a number of sessions. In the following excerpt, Eduardo, whom we met earlier, is introduced to the IFS model and guided toward accessing the self. In the process, he must unblend it from a "manager" part while negotiating with a "firefighter" to step aside. Subsequently, Eduardo's self is able to compassionately witness the manager part and perform a retrieval by letting the part know that it is present day and the risk of harm has passed.

Clinician: I want to introduce you to a model of therapy that we will use together. It is based on the idea that we all have a core self that embodies our essence and all of our finest qualities including calmness, curiosity, compassion, confidence, courage, clarity, connectedness, and creativity. We are born with these qualities; this is known as self-energy. However, we are also born with parts that help us to relate to and survive in the world. You have heard the language, "One part of me feels sad but another feels mad" or "On one hand I want this, but on the other I want that." It will be helpful to get to know these different parts of the mosaic mind. Some of these parts take on the role of protectors, keeping us safe from harm. They may do this in an outwardly positive way; for example, counteracting feelings of inadequacy by overworking and becoming perfectionistic. However, the fears of this part may cause anxiety, exhaustion, and a lack of belief in your own value. Other parts may protect you in ways that have a more negative effect. For example, a part may attempt to protect from painful thoughts or memories by using alcohol as a numbing agent. Though this can be used as a temporary way to avoid inner pain, the damage it causes to health, general well-being, and relationships is not helpful. Everyone has "parts" or facets of the self. All parts are welcome and all parts are in some way attempting to be helpful. In this model, we develop a way to communicate with all the various parts of you, finding a way to hear from them so that they can heal rather than be pushed away. Our goal is to get to know them better, to build their trust and understand their underlying hurts. When we heal, and unburden parts from their worries, they no longer feel the need to lead or be intense, because they begin to trust that you are now safe. Would you like to begin?

Eduardo: *Yes, I am interested in learning more.*

Clinician: You mentioned before that you have a particular part that seems to sabotage your relationships. Would you like to get to know this part better to see if we can help it?

Eduardo: *(nods) Yes, I'd like that.*

Clinician: How does this part show up?... Do you notice it in or around your body… Or perhaps visually?

Eduardo: *It's visual.*

Clinician: Can you tell me who and what you see?

Eduardo*: Yes, this part is the pacing detective. He looks pensive and highly anxious.*

Clinician: Are there words that go with this image?

Eduardo*: Yes, he is shouting and cursing. He is so stressed and has no control. He is fearful.*

Clinician: It sounds like this is a fearful part, what shall we call it?

(note: this is a manager)

Eduardo*: Yes, he is fearful…we can call it the fearful part for now.*

Clinician: How do you feel toward the fearful part?

Eduardo: I feel critical of this part. It's not a helpful response to have.

Clinician: It sounds like there's another part?

(note: this is a firefighter)

Eduardo: Yes, it's the teenager.

Clinician: Can you ask the critical part to step back/relax for a moment?

Eduardo: No, it doesn't want to step back.

Clinician: What is this part afraid would happen if it stepped back?

Eduardo: It would be too much to handle, possibly overwhelming.

Clinician: If we could take just a few minutes to get to know and hear from the critical part, would that be okay?

Eduardo: Yes.

Clinician: Thank you for creating the space to get to know this critical part. How do you feel toward this part?

Eduardo: It's been with me for a long time. It is fearful of getting hurt.

Clinician: Oh, I see… tell me more.

Eduardo: It doesn't want me to get hurt again.

Clinician: This part does not want you to get hurt again. How does this part serve you?

Eduardo: It protects me from pain.

Clinician: What will we call this part?

Eduardo: The protective part.

Clinician: How do you feel toward this protective part?

Eduardo: I appreciate it; I know it does not want me to be vulnerable or hurt.

Clinician: Would it feel okay to send this part a signal of your appreciation?

Eduardo: Yes.

Clinician: Is this part willing to give us permission to be with the fearful part?

Eduardo: Yes.

(Firefighter agrees to momentarily step back, consents to Eduardo connecting with Manager part)

Clinician: Okay. Take a moment to thank this protective part, letting it know you will listen for and appreciate its guidance…and then, when you are ready, you can connect with the fearful part.

Eduardo: Okay, this part feels more appreciated. I will listen for it more.

Clinician: How do you feel toward this fearful part?

Eduardo: I am interested in this part, but I don't like his energy – too much pacing. I don't really understand why?

Clinician: It sounds like you are curious to learn more about this part.

Eduardo: Yes, I am.

Clinician: Does this part know you are here with him?

Eduardo: No.

Clinician: How do you feel towards this part now?

Eduardo: I feel open but want to get to know him better.

Clinician: Would you like to send this part a signal of your curiosity, openness, and calmness?

Eduardo: Yes…I can do that.

Clinician: Does this part sense your presence?

Eduardo: Yes, but I am very far away.

Clinician: Would it be OK to get closer to the part?

Eduardo: Yes, I approached him and placed a hand on his shoulder. He turned around and we are making eye contact.

Clinician: What would you like to say to this part?

Eduardo: "We are safe. You don't need to be afraid anymore."

Clinician: Did he hear you?

Eduardo: Yes, he is taking that in.

Clinician: Can you ask this part what it fears will happen if you do not listen to it?

Eduardo: He is afraid that I will be vulnerable and hurt.

Clinician: That's understandable. There have been many times when you have been made to feel this way in the past.

Eduardo: Yes, there have been. He is the protector of a younger me.

(Note: The Manager is the protector of the Exile – the 6-year-old child)

Clinician: How do you feel toward this part?

Eduardo: Grateful: He protected me when no one else did.

Clinician: Do you want to share this gratitude toward this part?

Eduardo: Yes. He doesn't usually feel appreciated, so this feels good.

Clinician: What age is this part?

Eduardo: Fourteen.

Clinician: What age does this part think you are?

Eduardo: He thinks I'm in middle school.

Clinician: Do you want to tell this part about who you are now?

Eduardo: Yes. I am 32 now and I am strong, independent, and live in a peaceful home. I have security. I have choices. I am showing him what's been going on in my life since middle school. Things slowly got better. He is happy about that.

Clinician: Does this part have a response?

Eduardo: This part was so busy protecting me, he did not know that so much time had passed. This part has worked so hard. He is exhausted.

Clinician: Do you want to thank this part?

Eduardo: Thank you for being there for me, for protecting me. I have felt your presence all these years. This part is focused and powerful. I feel so appreciative of how hard he has worked.

Clinician: Can we hear from this part?

Eduardo: This part is relieved, but tired—very, very tired.

Clinician: I wonder if you would like to let this part know you appreciate its value, and that you will continue to visit it and build a relationship?

Eduardo: He would like that.

Clinician: If you like, maybe you could let this part know that you will be listening for its guidance.

Eduardo: Yes, that feels good and right – I will check in on him when I feel anxious or fearful.

Clinician: Let's take a moment to thank these parts for showing up today. In your own special and meaningful way, say goodbye to these parts, letting them know that you will continue to connect with and be curious about them.

Eduardo: Yes, that felt good.

Clinician: All parts are welcome and all parts are valuable. When we hear from these parts we may learn of their core beliefs, fears, and burdens, and in time perhaps negotiate with them to harmonize with us and have them unburden themselves.

Within IFS therapy, the clinician can begin to work toward achieving trauma resolution by recognizing parts and giving these parts a voice to express their needs within the internal family system. The objective is to support the client in developing an embodied sense of self that can compassionately hold all disparate emotions, vulnerable sensations, and young parts of self as they strive toward internal harmony (O'Shea Brown, 2020). The IFS concept of self-leadership provides a valuable language and positive resource when used as a therapy modality or used in conjunction with other therapeutic modalities.

Ordinarily the client is the gatekeeper of all internal communication; however, within IFS, there is a "direct access" technique that may need to be applied if there is considerable self-energy available in the client, alongside a protective part that is impeding the work (Schwartz, 2001). Direct access is an alternative approach to insight, wherein the clinician's "self" speaks directly to the client's "parts." Direct access can be accomplished as an explicit intervention or implicitly, if the clinician knows but does not reveal that they are speaking directly to the client's part. This technique must come from self-energy, or it will exacerbate mistrust (Schwartz & Sweezy, 2020). Therefore, the clinician must demonstrate the capacity to be aware of their own parts and how they may intervene during a session. Self-energy breeds self-energy, so this modality requires strong awareness of the clinician's own internal family. Additionally, clinicians must be mindful of their own affect, thought process, and countertransference (discussed further in Chap. 12). The IFS model depathologizes trauma-related splitting and empowers the client to be an active change agent in their own healing journey. By applying concepts and methods from the structure, strategies, and narrative of family therapy and sub-personalities, the IFS model provides a language necessary to understand one's parts and work through unresolved internal conflicts.

Summary

We were all once children, and still that inner child resides within us. But most adults are quite unaware of this. This lack of conscious relatedness to the inner child is precisely where so many emotional, behavioral, and relational difficulties stem from. A multi-consciousness approach to clinical treatment enables the trauma survivor to hear from the various parts of their own consciousness through a compassionate lens, which can ultimately pave the way for negotiation, clarity, and inner harmony. In the modalities of Eye Movement Desensitization and Reprocessing (EMDR) and IFS, there are opportunities for the trauma survivor to gently affirm or even rescue the younger self (O'Shea Brown, 2020). Akin to the IFS model, EMDR activates a healing process in many clients, in which scenes from the past are witnessed compassionately and younger parts of self are unburdened of feelings of guilt and shame (Twombly & Schwartz, 2008). The adult client is gently guided to hear from, protect, and even reparent their earlier self in a warm and nurturing way (Krauze & Gomez, 2013). This healing process creates a division between the past and present; it also creates an experience of releasing unexpressed anger, frustration, and pain in a safe and titrated way. Until the adult survivor of early trauma is taught to connect with and hear from the inner child, most survivors stumble through life, re-experiencing their pain through self-destructive behavior, traumatizing relationships (with similarly impaired partners), and a deep sense of shame. There are many ways to begin connecting and compassionately witnessing the inner child; however, it is strongly advised that you undertake training in an ego state modality, which will equip you as a clinician and enable the client to go deeper in a safe and controlled manner. Information on training in Internal Family Systems (IFS) therapy is listed in the Appendix.

Questions and Activities for Discussion and Further Reflection

1. Private assignment: Write a letter to your younger self through loving eyes as a compassionate supportive adult.
2. Watch the movie "Inside Out," and write a one-page reflection on how it feels to think about yourself as "parts" of a mosaic mind.
3. Have an open discussion on whether you would be interested in advancing your knowledge in ego states through training or certification. If yes, what attracts you to the intervention? Do you anticipate any barriers or challenges to doing this work?

Acknowledgments Elizabeth Janssen, NP, a psychiatric nurse practitioner and psychoanalyst, contributed richly to this chapter through her insights on the IFS model and psychoanalytic theory. She is certified in IFS, is an EMDRIA-certified consultant and therapist, and maintains a private practice in New York City.

References

Fraser, G. (1991). The dissociative table technique: A strategy for working with ego states and dissociative disorders and ego-state therapy. *Dissociation, 4*(4), 205–213.

Janet, P. (1889). *L'Automatisme psychologique*. Paris: Felix Alcan. (Reprint: Paris, Société Pierre Janet, 1973).

Jung, C. G. (1958). The psychology of the child archetype. In V. deLasco (Ed.), *Psyche and symbol* (pp. 113–131). New York, NY: Doubleday. (Original work published 1940).

Krauze, P. K., & Gomez, A. M. (2013). EMDR therapy and the use of internal family systems strategies with children. In C. Forgash & M. Copeley (Eds.), *Healing the heart of trauma and dissociation with EMDR and ego state therapy* (pp. 295–311). New York, NY: Springer.

O'Shea Brown, G. (2020). Internal family systems informed eye movement desensitization and reprocessing: An integrative technique for treatment of complex posttraumatic stress disorder. *International Body Psychotherapy Journal, 19*(2).

O'Shea Brown, G. (2021). Reflections on providing virtual eye movement desensitization and reprocessing therapy in the wake of COVID-19: Survival through adaptation. In C. Tosone (Ed.), *Shared trauma, shared resilience during a pandemic: Social work in the time of COVID-19*. Cham, Switzerland: Springer.

Perls, F. (1973). *The Gestalt approach & eye witness to therapy*. Ben Lomond, CA: Science & Behavior Books.

Schwartz, R. (1995). *Internal family systems therapy*. New York, NY: Guilford Press.

Schwartz, R. (2001). *Introduction to the internal family systems model*. Oak Park, IL: Trailhead Publications.

Schwartz, R., & Sweezy, M. (2020). *Internal family systems therapy* (2nd ed.). New York, NY: Guilford Press.

Siegel, D. J. (1999). *The developing mind: toward a neurobiology of interpersonal experience*. New York, NY: Guilford Press.

Twombly, J. H., & Schwartz, R. C. (2008). The integration of the internal family systems model and EMDR. In C. Forgash & M. Copeley (Eds.), *Healing the heart of trauma and dissociation with EMDR and ego state therapy* (pp. 295–311). New York, NY: Springer.

van der Hart, O., Nijenhuis, E., & Steele, K. (2006). *The haunted self: Structural dissociation and the treatment of chronic traumatization*. New York, NY: Norton.

van Der Hart, O., Nijenhuis, E., Steele, K., & Brown, D. (2004). Trauma-related dissociation: conceptual clarity lost and found. *Australian and New Zealand Journal of Psychiatry, 38*, 906–914. https://doi.org/10.1111/j.1440-1614.2004.01480.x

van der Hart, O., Nijenhuis, E. R. S., & Solomon, R. (2010). Dissociation of the personality in complex trauma-related disorders and EMDR: Theoretical considerations. *Journal of EMDR Practice and Research, 4*(2), 76–92. https://doi.org/10.1891/1933-3196.4.2.76

van der Hart, O., Steele, K., Boon, S., & Brown, P. (1993). The treatment of traumatic memories: Synthesis, realization and integration. *Dissociation, 6*, 162–180.

Watkins, J., & Watkins, H. (1997). *Ego States: Theory and Therapy*. New York: W.W. Norton.

Chapter 10
Turning Wounds into Wisdom: Resilience and Posttraumatic Growth

Through my observations of my clients, I have witnessed the undeniable power of resilience, that is, the ability that humans have to adapt to, navigate, and even grow from life's most painful events. Resilience has been described by Garmezy (1993) as the capacity to adapt successfully to disturbances that threaten functioning, sustainability, and future development. Therefore, resilience is not the absence of suffering but the capacity to adapt to survive in painful or unpredictable circumstances. Researchers have even argued that survival through hardship and triumph over adversity can make a survivor more focused and more feeling and, in turn, expand one's capacity for compassion, spirituality, and creativity (Garmezy & Masten, 1986; Miller, 1997; Sapienza & Masten, 2011; Scheff, 2003). Thus, survival through adaption and healing from trauma can be seen not just as a triumph over adversity but also as a personal evolution. This chapter begins with an exploration of vulnerability and shame through the lens of Shame Resilience Theory, developed by Brown (2006). Subsequently, the anatomy of resilience will be explored through a theoretical and clinical lens. Finally, this chapter will explore the emergence and impact of the Posttraumatic Growth Model and the impact this has on an individual's intuition, internal guidance, and power.

Vulnerability and Shame

We have all experienced shame at one time or another; however, the painful emotion of shame is rarely spoken about, even in close, intimate relationships. Most people feel compelled to suppress this emotion or deny its very existence. Shame-based cognition is often suppressed and can manifest in harmful behaviors (Herman, 1992). Brené Brown, PhD, LMSW, has helped lift this veil of secrecy, initially through her 2011 TED Talk entitled "The Power of Vulnerability." At the time of writing, it has garnered over 13 million views online and opened up a global

G. O'Shea Brown, *Healing Complex Posttraumatic Stress Disorder*, Essential Clinical Social Work Series, https://doi.org/10.1007/978-3-030-61416-4_10

discussion on the importance of embracing shame and vulnerability. The theory emerging from Brown's qualitative research is termed Shame Resilience Theory (SRT) (2006). Defining shame as a painful emotion derived from a belief that one is unworthy of acceptance or belonging (Brown, 2006), Brown differentiates the experience of shame from that of guilt. Shame centers on "self" rather than behavior. Shame can lead to the cognition "I am bad," whereas guilt leads to the cognition "I did something bad." In this light, guilt is viewed as an adaptive and helpful emotion, as it is an acknowledgment that your thoughts or behaviors do not align with your values. This misalignment with the moral compass creates psychological discomfort, which in turn can serve as a catalyst for positive change. Brown (2006) argues that it may even lead to a "personal awakening," in which you identify the necessary adaptations required to achieve homeostasis.

Shame, on the other hand, can be detrimental to growth and expression. Within the SRT model, it is posited that shame is a psycho-social-cultural construct. The psychological component consists of an individual's emotions, thoughts, and behaviors related to their sense of self. The social component involves interpersonal relationships and the need for connection. The cultural component is linked to societal expectations and the pressure to be accepted. Brown (2006) elaborates that shame is exacerbated by secrecy, silence, and judgment and is associated with the feelings of being trapped, powerless, or isolated. Societal pressures often drive individuals to portray a flawless or seemingly perfect self, thus masking inner subjectivity and vulnerability. This masking only succeeds in alienating us from ourselves and others. In the famous words of T.S. Eliot (1915) in his poem, *The Love Song of J. Alfred Prufrock*, you may feel compelled "to prepare a face to meet the faces that you meet." Perpetually doing so robs us of any chance to feel completely accepted, seen, or compassionately witnessed in moments of imperfection and vulnerability. It also serves to heighten feelings of being trapped, isolated, or powerless.

Shame is often an interpersonally driven emotion, stemming from altruism and fear of harming others (Baumeister & Leary, 1995; Baumeister, Stillwell, & Heatherton, 1994; Gilbert, Pehl, & Allan, 1994; Zahn-Waxler, Kochanska, McKnew, & Krupnik, 1990). The development of conscience, of which guilt is the manifestation, is tied to a deep fear of not belonging, not being accepted, and possibly becoming an outcast. The SRT model postulates that empathy is the antidote for shame. Brown (2006) states that opportunities to experience empathy through connection and empowerment counteract feelings of being trapped, powerless, and isolated and facilitate freedom from shame. To put it colloquially, showing our vulnerability to trustworthy, responsive others allows us to connect in a way that is absent of secrecy, silence, and judgment. When you allow yourself to be vulnerable, you can become open with yourself and others. Brown teaches that vulnerability is the birthplace of innovation, creativity, and change. With the absence of shame comes strength, courage, and resilience.

The Anatomy of Resilience

When a client privileges you with their pain, this is a sign of healing. When a client shows up each week, courageous, open, and willing, this is a sign of healing. When a client advocates that they are feeling unsafe or untrusting of the process, this, too, is a sign of healing. Healing is an ever-unfolding process of evolution, vulnerability, and self-compassion. Healing is a continuous process of learning to choose: choosing yourself, choosing a better life, and, most importantly, choosing self-care over self-destruction. Healing is a process of unburdening, becoming more yourself, and becoming more than you could have ever hoped for in your darkest and most ominous moments. In the words of Herman (1992), "the resolution of the trauma is never final; recovery is never complete" (p.152). The impact of past traumatic events may be awakened at particular points, despite being sufficiently resolved at one stage of recovery in the life cycle. Though we as clinicians cannot take the pain away, we can take that walk with the survivor, serving as their empathic witness and guide as they work to overcome these milestones in the healing journey (O'Shea Brown, 2021). However, as clinicians we should also be interested in understanding what sparks this journey. What is it that drives certain individuals to work through, process, and even heal from the deep wounds of trauma?

We live in an age with multiple, often overwhelming complex challenges. At the time of this publication, there is large-scale displacement and uncertainty due to a global pandemic, and the prospect of much more of the same resulting from climate change, along with a human rights movement playing out on a global scale. These forces are shaping a world in which resilience will be more important than ever. The word "resilience" derives from the Latin word meaning to rebound (Brown, 2006). Within systems theory, it can be defined as the capacity of a system to absorb disturbance and re-organize while undergoing change in order to retain continuity in function, structure, and identity (Walker, Holling, Carpenter, & Kinzig, 2004). In the context of exposure to significant adversity, resilience is measured by our capacity to navigate and negotiate for the resources that we need in order to survive. Masten and Wright (1998) describe resiliency as a pattern of positive adaptation in the context of past or present adversity. This echoes the work of Stanton-Salazar and Spina (2000), who associate resilience with the acquisition of a necessary set of inner resources, social competencies, and cultural strategies that enable individuals to not only survive but recover or even thrive after stressful events. However, necessity is indeed the mother of invention. No one chooses to become strong or resilient; it is rather a quality imposed upon a person cruelly, by force.

We must remember, at the same time, that it is rare for individuals never to be confronted with adversity or challenging circumstances during the course of a lifetime (Masten, 2012). Adversity is more prevalent than we would like to admit. As discussed in Chap. 4, the Adverse Childhood Experiences Study (ACES) found that 67% percent of the population has endured at least one ACE, while 12.6% have endured four or more ACEs (Felitti et al., 1998). While it is upsetting to contemplate such large numbers of children experiencing significant adversity, such numbers make it possible for child development researchers to investigate why some children navigate disadvantage and adversity better than others. The scientific study of resilience is a relatively new area of investigation, which began with questions about why some at-risk children and youth somehow defy the odds and thrive (Garmezy, Masten, & Tellegen, 1984; Luthar, Cicchetti, & Becker, 2000; Rutter, 2013). In recent years, resilience research has expanded its focus to include survivors of stress and trauma across the lifespan (Southwick, Litz, Charney, & Friedman, 2011).

The National Scientific Council on the Developing Child (2015) found that resilience is a highly interactive process between individual characteristics and the person's connection with their environment. Looking at well-adapted children from disadvantaged backgrounds (i.e., those who did better than others), they found that individual children were more likely to be resilient if they had access to internal and external protective factors to buffer the effects of adversity. Individual qualities which served as protective factors included confidence in their ability to control their own lives and futures, skill building, intelligence, problem-solving abilities, forward thinking, and, most importantly, the capacity to consider consequences before action (Garmezy, 1981; Haggerty, Sherrod, Garmezy, & Rutter, 1994; Luthar & Brown, 2007; Masten, 2007; Rutter, 2012). External protective factors included access to networks of support and relationships to others (Holling, 1973; Masten, 2007; Shonkoff, Richter, van der Gaag, & Bhutta, 2012; Wu et al., 2013). It is worth noting that individual qualities also predispose children either to have or to not have good relationships with others: Such relationships require qualities of empathy, expressiveness, warmth, and sociability (Masten, 2001). Therefore, resiliency can be dependent on one's capacity to ask for help and to access trusting relationships to rely upon in times of crisis.

These internal and external protective factors buffer the effects of adversity. Without protective factors, individuals are more likely to employ or experience maladaptive coping mechanisms such as substance abuse, minimizing of self-worth, or an increase in risky behaviors (Rutter, 2012). In order to promote resilience in the individual, it is important to consider a systems perspective in that individuals are embedded in families, communities, societies and cultures, and organizations. Thus, interventions targeted at any one of these levels will affect other levels. Whether that concerns positive meaningful change or disequilibrium, the system impacts overall resiliency. Hobfall and colleagues (Hobfoll et al., 2007) identified empirically supported intervention principles to be used as guidelines for individuals impacted by mass violence and natural disaster. These principles discussed immediate- to mid-term care following a traumatic life event. At the level of community, interventions to enhance resilience typically require integrated educational and training programs that involve a diverse group of experts, systems, and community members (Norris, Stevens, Pfefferbaum, Wyche, & Pfefferbaum, 2008). This sense of community-fostered connection and compassionate witnessing, in turn, creates opportunities for survivors to be vulnerable, heard, and supported. Interventions designed to enhance resilience can be directed at individuals of all ages and can be employed before, during, or after stressful and traumatic life events.

With every adversity that is overcome, an individual builds self-belief and a sense of trust in their own capacity, and this can build a sense of mastery. With triumph over adversity, there is an experience of successfully overcoming a stressful event that can promote coping skills and strategies that an individual carries forward. Garmezy (1981) has referred to this as the "steeling effect," by which certain moderate stressors will enhance coping skills and foster resilience. Having come to terms with the setback and adapted to survive, the individual now has an internal guiding voice that proclaims, "If you got through this you can get through anything" or "I know I have it in me to get through this." Stanton-Salazar and Spina (2000) assert that an individual's resilience is also determined by their capacity to reflectively draw from the experience to enhance subsequent functioning. After adversity has passed and newly created homeostasis emerges, the individual can now venture forth with a sense of empowerment and trust in their connection to their internal guiding voice.

Posttraumatic Growth Model

As counterintuitive as it may sound, from tragedy and trauma can come opportunity. The loss of stability and security allows room for growth, adaption, and evolution. The Posttraumatic Growth Model, hereafter PG, posits that in the aftermath of trauma and the return to homeostasis, development of a positive outlook on life can emerge (Tedeschi & Calhoun, 1996; Tedeschi & Calhoun, 2004). Fredrickson & Losada, (2005) argue that trauma creates a need for growth to aid survival and with this develops a greater capacity to find positive meaning in the face of adversity. PG can lead to positive changes in the way an individual relates to others, increased openness to possibilities, and strengthened belief in one's ability to adapt and control outcomes, in addition to deepening spirituality, creativity, and appreciation for life (Tedeschi & Calhoun, 2004; Tedeschi, Calhoun, & Cann, 2007).

Ultimately, the trauma causes a massive deviation in one's life, which can serve as an opportunity to break old patterns. This creates opportunity for change and may even prompt enhanced accountability and a serious life review, as a survivor attempts to navigate a new way forward. Research has shown a positive correlation between posttraumatic stress disorder and PG, suggesting that a strong negative reaction to trauma is correlated with an eventual capacity to make positive changes based on that trauma; furthermore, it is suggested that the highest growth levels stem from exposure to grave adversity, e.g., life-threatening experiences (Tedeschi & Calhoun, 1996; Tedeschi & Calhoun, 2004; Linley & Joseph, 2004). In this scenario, the survivor can view their situation through the lens of fear and loss or as a realm of possibility and progress; in reality, it can be both. PG is often the result of an individual having taken a journey of realignment, reprioritization, and rebuilding in their emotional connections, physical health, and environment after a trauma. Even after PTSD has developed, relief and personal growth can occur. PG is more likely to happen, if individual survivors receive trauma-informed therapy and have close supportive relationships (Tedeschi & Calhoun, 1996; Tedeschi & Calhoun, 2004; Linley & Joseph, 2004). In the task of healing, therefore, each survivor must find a way to restore a sense of connection with the wider community in order to discover some meaning in their experience that transcends the limits of personal tragedy.

Researchers have even argued that survival through hardship and triumph over adversity can make a survivor more focused and more feeling and, in turn, expand one's capacity for compassion, spirituality, and creativity (Garmezy & Masten, 1986; Werner & Smith, 1992; Miller, 1997; Sapienza & Masten, 2011; Scheff, 2003). Thus, survival through adaption and healing from trauma can be seen not just as a triumph over adversity but also as a personal evolution. I was deeply moved by the resilience and adaptability I observed in my clients at my trauma-focused practice in the wake of the COVID-19 pandemic. Despite—or pointedly, perhaps because of—having encountered so much past adversity, hardship, and suffering, these clients were largely well-equipped to harness their inner strengths and resources to rebound quickly from setbacks resulting from the pandemic. When the crisis hit, many were deep into their methodical, solution-focused mindset and accordingly began to strategize, pivot, and make decisive choices. There was a notable shift away from the anticipatory anxiety many had reported feeling pervasively throughout their lives to a place of decisive action. When I verbalized my admiration, the same response came back to me time and time again—"I know I have it in me to get through this, as I have faced much worse before and came out with a deep trust in myself, feeling even stronger and more capable than before." An inner trust and innate wisdom had been built through past experiences of distress and recovery.

Summary

Resilience has been described as the capacity to adapt successfully to disturbances that threaten functioning, sustainability, and future development. Therefore, resilience is not the absence of suffering but the capacity to adapt to survive in painful or even unpredictable circumstances. Within Shame Resilience Theory (SRT), it is posited that shame is a psycho-social-cultural construct. The psychological component of shame centers on an individual's emotions, thoughts, and behaviors related to their sense of self. The social component of shame involves interpersonal relationships and the need for connection. The cultural component is linked to societal expectations and the pressure to be accepted. Shame is inflamed by secrecy, silence, and judgment and is associated with the feelings of being trapped, powerless, or isolated.

The SRT model also postulates that empathy is the antidote of shame. Vulnerability is the birthplace of innovation, creativity, and change and the path to freedom from shame. With the absence of shame comes strength, courage, and resilience. Resilience is the focus of the Posttraumatic Growth Model, which posits that in the aftermath of trauma and the return to homeostasis, development of a positive outlook on life can emerge (Tedeschi & Calhoun, 1996; Tedeschi & Calhoun, 2004).

Researchers have even argued that survival through hardship and triumph over adversity can make a survivor more focused and more feeling, in turn expanding their capacity for compassion, spirituality, and creativity (Garmezy & Masten, 1986; Miller, 1997; Sapienza & Masten, 2011; Scheff, 2003). Thus, survival through adaption and healing from trauma can be seen not just as a triumph over adversity but also as a personal evolution.

Questions and Activities for Discussion and Further Reflection

1. Assignment Suggestion: Report a case study of an individual you have worked with. Assess how Shame Resilience Theory informed your work, assessment, and clinical treatment.
2. How is shame different from guilt, according to SRT?
3. Can you define the following terms: (i) resilience, (ii) posttraumatic growth, and (iii) protective factors?
4. Have an open discussion on whether you believe resiliency is impacted by poverty, intersectionality, ethnicity, and immigration status.

References

Baumeister, F., Stillwell, M., & Heatherton, F. (1994). Guilt: An interpersonal approach. *Psychological Bulletin, 115*, 243–267.

Baumeister, R., & Leary, R. (1995). The need to belong: Desire for interpersonal attachments as a fundamental human motivation. *Psychological Bulletin, 17*(3), 497–529.

Brown, B. (2006). Shame resilience theory: A grounded theory of women and shame. *Families in Society, 87*(01).

Eliot, T. S. (1915) The love song of J. Alfred Prufrock. *Poetry: A Magazine of Verse,* June 1915, pp. 130–135.

Felitti, V. J., Anda, R. F., Nordenberg, D., Williamson, D. F., Spitz, A. M., Edwards, V., ... Marks, J. S. (1998). Relationship of childhood abuse and household dysfunction to many of the leading causes of death in adults. The adverse childhood experiences (ACE) study. *American Journal of Preventive Medicine, 14*, 245–258.

Fredrickson, B. L., & Losada, M. F. (2005). Positive Affect and the Complex Dynamics of Human Flourishing. *American Psychologist, 60*(7), 678–686. https://doi.org/10.1037/0003-066X.60.7.678

Garmezy, N. (1981). Children under stress: Perspectives on antecedents and correlates of vulnerability and resistance to psychopathology. In A. I. Rabin, J. Aronoff, A. M. Barclay, & R. A. Zucker (Eds.), *Further explorations in personality* (pp. 196–269). New York, NY: Wiley.

Garmezy, N. (1993). Vulnerability and resilience. In D. C. Funder, R. D. Parke, et al. (Eds.), *Studying lives through time: Personality and development* (pp. 377–398). Washington, DC: American Psychological Association.

Garmezy, N., & Masten, A. S. (1986). Stress, competence, and resilience: Common frontiers for therapist and psychopathologist. *Behavior Therapy, 17*(5), 500.

Garmezy, N., Masten, A. S., & Tellegen, A. (1984). The study of stress and competence in children: A building block for developmental psychopathology. *Child Development, 55*, 97–111. http://www.jstor.org/stable/1129837

Gilbert, P., Pehl, J., & Allan, S. (1994). The phenomenology of shame and guilt: An empirical investigation. *British Journal of Medical Psychology, 67*, 23–36.

Haggerty, R. J., Sherrod, L. R., Garmezy, N., & Rutter, M. (Eds.). (1994). *Stress, risk, and resilience in children and adolescents: Processes, mechanisms, and interventions*. Cambridge, UK: Cambridge University Press.

Herman, J. L. (1992). *Trauma and recovery: The aftermath of violence*. New York, NY: Basic Books.

Hobfoll, S. E., Watson, P., Bell, C. C., Bryant, R. A., Brymer, M. J., Friedman, M. J., et al. (2007). Five essential elements of immediate and mid-term mass trauma intervention: Empirical evidence. *Psychiatry, 70*, 283–315. https://doi.org/10.1521/psyc.2007.70.4.283

Holling, C. S. (1973). Resilience and stability of ecological systems. *Annual Review of Ecology and Systematics, 4*, 1–23.

Linley, P. A., & Joseph, S. (2004). Positive change following trauma and adversity: a review. *Journal of traumatic stress, 17*(1), 11–21. https://doi.org/10.1023/B:JOTS.0000014671.27856.7e

Luthar, S. S., & Brown, P. J. (2007). Maximizing resilience through diverse levels of inquiry: Prevailing paradigms, possibilities, and priorities for the future. *Development and Psychopathology, 19*(3), 931–955.

Luthar, S. S., Cicchetti, D., & Becker, B. (2000). The construct of resilience: A critical evaluation and guidelines for future work. *Child Development, 71*, 543–562. https://doi.org/10.1111/1467-8624.00164

Masten, A. S. (2001). Ordinary magic: Resilience processes in development. *The American Psychologist, 56*, 227–238.

Masten, A. S. (2007). Resilience in developing systems: Progress and promise as the fourth wave rises. *Development and Psychopathology, 19*(3), 921–930.

Masten, A. S. (2012). Risk and resilience in development. In P. D. Zelazo (Ed.), *The Oxford handbook of developmental psychology* (Vol. 2). New York, NY: Oxford University Press.

Masten, A. S., & Wright, M. O. (1998). Cumulative risk and protection models of child maltreatment. *Journal of Aggression, Maltreatment & Trauma, 2*(1), 7–30.

Miller, A. (1997). *The drama of the gifted child: The search for the true self*. New York, NY: Basic Books.

National Scientific Council on the Developing ChildChildren. (2015). *Supportive relationships and active skill-building strengthen the foundations of resilience* (Working paper no. 13). Retrieved from http://www.developingchild.harvard.edu

Norris, F. H., Stevens, S. P., Pfefferbaum, B., Wyche, K. F., & Pfefferbaum, R. L. (2008). Community resilience as a metaphor, theory, set of capacities, and strategy for disaster readiness. *American Journal of Community Psychology, 41*, 127–150. https://doi.org/10.1007/s10464-007-9156-6

O'Shea Brown, G. (2021). Reflections on providing virtual eye movement desensitization and reprocessing therapy in the wake of COVID-19: Survival through adaptation. In C. Tosone (Ed.), *Shared trauma, shared resilience during a pandemic: Social work in the time of COVID-19*. Cham, Switzerland: Springer.

Rutter, M. (2012). Resilience as a dynamic concept. *Development and Psychopathology, 24*(2), 335–344.

Rutter, M. (2013). Annual research review: Resilience – Clinical implications. *Journal of Child Psychology and Psychiatry, 54*, 474–487. https://doi.org/10.1111/j.1469-7610.2012.02615.x

Sapienza, J. K., & Masten, A. S. (2011). Understanding and promoting resilience in children and youth. *Current Opinion in Psychiatry, 24*(4), 267–273. https://doi.org/10.1097/YCO.0b013e32834776a8

Scheff, T. (2003). Shame in self and society. *Symbolic Interaction, 26*, 239–262.

Shonkoff, J. P., Richter, L., van der Gaag, J., & Bhutta, Z. A. (2012). An integrated scientific framework for child survival and early childhood development. *Pediatrics, 129*(2), e460–e472. https://doi.org/10.1542/peds.2011-0366

Southwick, S. M., Litz, B. T., Charney, D., & Friedman, M. J. (Eds.). (2011). *Resilience and mental health: Challenges across the lifespan*. Cambridge, UK: Cambridge Press. https://doi.org/10.1017/CBO9780511994791

Stanton-Salazar, R. D., & Spina, S. U. (2000). The network orientations of highly resilient urban minority youth: A network-analytic account of minority socialization and its educational implications. *The Urban Review, 32*, 227–261. https://doi.org/10.1023/A:1005122211864

Tedeschi, R. G., & Calhoun, L. G. (1996). The posttraumatic growth inventory: Measuring the positive legacy of trauma. *Journal of Traumatic Stress, 9*, 455–471.

Tedeschi, R. G., & Calhoun, L. G. (2004). Posttraumatic growth: Conceptual foundations and empirical evidence. *Psychological Inquiry, 15*, 1–18.

Tedeschi, R. G., Calhoun, L. G., & Cann, A. (2007). Evaluating resource gain: Understanding and misunderstanding posttraumatic growth. *Applied Psychology-an International Review-Psychologie Appliquee-Revue Internationale, 56*, 396–406.

Walker, B., Holling, C. S., Carpenter, S. R., & Kinzig, A. (2004). Resilience, adaptability and transformability in social-ecological systems. *Ecology and Society, 9*(2), 5–13.

Werner, E. E., & Smith, R. S. (1992). *Overcoming the odds: High risk children from birth to adulthood.* Ithaca, NY: Cornell University Press.

Wu, G., Feder, A., Cohen, H., Kim, J. J., Calderon, S., Charney, D. S., & Mathé, A. A. (2013). Understanding resilience. *Frontiers in Behavioral Neuroscience, 7*, 10. https://doi.org/10.3389/fnbeh.2013.00010

Zahn-Waxler, C., Kochanska, G., McKnew, D., & Krupnik, J. (1990). Patterns of guilt in children of depressed and well mothers. *Developmental Psychology, 26*, 51–59.

Chapter 11
Vicarious Trauma and Professional Self-Care for the Trauma Clinician

Shared trauma in the wake of a global pandemic has created a unique bond between the clinician and the client. While navigating one's own fears, anxieties, and losses, the clinician must also serve as an anchor to the client in an unsteady and unpredictable world. The profound impact of collective catastrophic events can create immense hardship for clinicians living and working in traumatogenic environments. Even outside of the pandemic, clinicians who specialize in the treatment of trauma and complex trauma have a distinct susceptibility to vicarious trauma (VT) due to the repeated exposure to the harrowing details of their clients' traumatic experiences. VT refers to the experience of indirect trauma such as the clinicians' continuous emotional engagement with a clients' traumatic material. This can create cognitive distortions and changes in core belief systems of the clinician, which, in turn, can adversely impact overall functioning and emotional well-being. Many clinicians enter into the profession to compassionately witness, heal, and affirm their clients due to their own lived experiences of trauma. Without adequate use of clinical supervision, professional boundaries, and self-care, repeated exposure to trauma can be precarious to the clinician's well-being, causing retraumatization or compassion fatigue. This chapter will provide a conceptualization of VT before exploring how this may impact upon the clinician and the therapeutic alliance. Secondly, this chapter will review the impact of countertransference before proposing strategies to effectively manage its adverse effects. Finally, this chapter will explore the role of professional supervision and the importance of self-care for the trauma clinician.

Conceptualization of Vicarious Trauma

The terms secondary traumatic stress (STS) and vicarious trauma (VT) are often used to describe the experience of indirect trauma, that is, the experience that can occur when a clinician is continuously engaged with or overly exposed to clients'

G. O'Shea Brown, *Healing Complex Posttraumatic Stress Disorder*, Essential Clinical Social Work Series, https://doi.org/10.1007/978-3-030-61416-4_11

traumatic material over a prolonged period of time. Charles Figley, PhD, described STS as a secondary trauma that results from indirect exposure to trauma. Figley (1995) argued that STS is a natural consequence of becoming knowledgeable of a trauma having occurred and experiencing the stress of wanting to help and cease suffering for the survivor. STS can lead to many adverse side effects for the clinician including but not limited to cynicism, lethargy, irritability, reduced productivity, feelings of hopelessness, anger, despair, feelings of re-experiencing of the event, nightmares, and anxiety, in addition to avoidance of people or activities (Siegfried, 2008). Stamm, Varra, Pearlman, and Giller (2002) attributes professional isolation (i.e., lack of peer support and clinical supervision), larger caseloads, and frequent contact with traumatized people as potential risks for the development of STS. Over a lengthy period of time, this could adversely impact the clinician's health, well-being, and overall job satisfaction.

The term *vicarious traumatization* was coined by Pearlman and Saakvitne (1995). It is utilized to describe the profound shift in worldview that can occur when clinicians are working with and are continuously exposed to the painful stories of trauma survivors. Vicarious traumatization is characterized by a change in core beliefs and fundamental viewpoints about the world, which are altered or damaged due to overexposure to traumatic material. A clinician impacted by vicarious traumatization may experience a loss of trust, a sense of hypervigilance, and a changed view of the world and the people around them. For instance, a clinician who works with survivors of recent and retrospective child abuse may begin to lose trust in all individuals who approach their own children due to the long-term cumulative impact of traumatic stress to which they have been exposed. There are many potential adverse effects of vicarious traumatization for clinicians including professional burnout, compassion fatigue, and possibly retraumatization of their own histories. Situations that increase the risk of vicarious trauma for a clinician may include:

- A clinician working in forensic assessment who frequently reads graphic reports and views disturbing images.
- A clinician hearing a detailed traumatic story over a prolonged period of time.
- A clinician working with individuals who have experienced a similar trauma to the clinician. For instance, a clinician who is the survivor of child sexual abuse decides to work with fellow survivors professionally in adulthood.
- A clinician working with domestic violence survivors loses hope that healthy relationships and boundaries are possible.
- A clinician who has frequent or chronic exposure to emotional and detailed accounts by children of traumatic events.
- A clinician attending a court hearing or conference where disturbing images and details are described or shown over a prolonged period of time.

In order for a clinician to understand their reactions to the clients' trauma narratives, self-awareness can be fostered preferably through self-analysis in psychotherapy in addition to continuous use of clinical supervision (O'Shea Brown, 2021). This was crucial in the wake of COVID-19, a time of practice innovation and shared trauma. The term shared trauma refers to the clinician's experience of living and practicing in traumatogenic environments while striving to provide effective professional services despite being exposed to the same collective trauma in their personal lives (Altman & Davies, 2002; Eidelson, D'Alessio, & Eidelson, 2003; Saakvitne, 2002; Tosone, 2006; Tosone et al., 2003; Tosone & Bialkin, 2003). Shared trauma, as described by Tosone, Nuttman-Shwartz, and Stephens (2012), refers to the affective, behavioral, cognitive, spiritual, and multimodal responses that clinicians experience as a result of dual exposure to the same collective trauma as their clients. This can impact a clinician personally and professionally in the clinical dyad; therefore, awareness of countertransference is of the utmost importance. The precipitous unfolding of COVID-19 has caused many rapid changes in the provision of psychotherapy; most notably, telepsychotherapy has suddenly become a necessary clinical practice adaptation where it had recently represented an emerging clinical trend. Furthermore, shared trauma in the wake of a global pandemic has created a unique bond between the clinician and the client. Research assessing the profound impact that COVID-19 created for clinicians living and working in an uncertain time is ongoing at the time of this publication. However, recent research has indicated that this has been a period of increased risk of vicarious traumatization for many mental health professionals.

Aafjes-van Doorn, Békés, Prout, and Hoffman (2020) conducted qualitative research into psychotherapists' vicarious traumatization during the COVID-19 pandemic. The study had a sample group comprised of 339 clinicians who were surveyed about their professional practices and experiences during the pandemic. Results demonstrated that levels of vicarious traumatization were common among all members of the sample group, with 15% reporting heightened levels of vicarious traumatization. Clinicians most at risk of vicarious traumatization were found to be younger and earlier in their career path (with less clinical experience). Those reporting symptoms of vicarious traumatization expressed that they had faced negative online treatment experiences such as feeling more distressed, tired, less competent, and less confident in their clinical ability. Other aversive clinical experiences included feeling less connected with the client and having a weaker therapeutic alliance than before, which were also associated with higher levels of vicarious traumatization. A loss of peer support and a professional camaraderie were also identified as complicating factors to professional well-being. Aafjes-van Doorn et al. (2020) strongly recommended the provision of personal and professional support for clinicians working remotely amid a shared trauma.

Understanding Countertransference and Compassion Fatigue

The term countertransference is often mistakenly used interchangeably with secondary trauma. In order to avoid such confusion, it is first necessary to define and explain the difference between the respective terms. Tosone et al. (2012) state that countertransference refers only to the clinician's affective responses toward the client in the therapeutic dyad, while secondary trauma relates to consequences and changes in the clinician's personal life. Courtois (2010) cautions that trauma survivors may unconsciously induce clinicians into a reenactment of their trauma, provoking polarizing countertransference responses. When the nature of the original trauma is human-induced or perhaps even perpetrated by a family member, this compromises a survivor's ability to trust relationally and develop a positive self-concept. Consequently, it is natural and self-protective for survivors to be mistrustful or even suspicious of others. Courtois (2010) cautions that survivors of trauma may be especially vigilant regarding issues pertaining to confidentiality due to their past history of intrusion or violation. For survivors of trauma, vigilance regarding confidentiality has the potential to reawaken fear and mistrust. This can serve as a catalyst, slowing the time it takes to form an effective therapeutic alliance.

Braun (1986) cautions that the clinician must be mindful and conscientious not to respond defensively to this perceived intentional affront but rather compassionately witness this behavior in order to prevent retraumatization. Trust is built gradually over time through small consistent acts of reliance, responsivity, and connection. To earn the privilege of the survivor's trust, the clinician must continuously demonstrate trustworthiness, compassion, and honesty. The cumulative effect of being confronted with more suffering than one is able to ameliorate can cause compassion fatigue. According to Figley (1995), compassion fatigue refers to reactions that emerge from the trauma clinician's overexposure to client suffering over extended periods of time. Absorbing and compassionately witnessing the emotional weight of the trauma survivor's experiences can, over time, negatively impact both the professional identity and personal life of the trauma clinician.

Figley (2002) notes that the trauma clinician may, over time, notice changes in their emotions, cognitions, and behavior due to compassion fatigue. In terms of cognition, compassion fatigue may include the therapist's lowered concentration, decreased self-esteem, apathy, negativity, depersonalization, thoughts of harm to the self or others, and preoccupation with the trauma (Berzoff & Kita, 2010). In terms of emotional changes, the trauma clinician may experience feelings of powerlessness, guilt, rage, fear, survivor's guilt, depression, and depletion. Finally, in terms of behavioral changes, the trauma clinician may exhibit impatience, irritation, sadness, moodiness, sleep disturbances, nightmares, hypervigilance, accident proneness, and losing things (Berzoff & Kita, 2010; Figley, 2002). Compassion fatigue can negatively impact the clinician and the client. However, we must remember that compassion does not always result in fatigue; hence, being mindful of the risk and engaged with the correct supports is vital.

The importance of professional self-care and ongoing supervision is discussed later in this chapter.

The Role of Clinical Supervision and Professional Self-Care

In managing any countertransference, gaining awareness of one's own internal processing is paramount, specifically in relation to shared trauma. If unnoticed, countertransference and VT can lead to ethical dilemmas in the clinical dyad pertaining to self-disclosure, professional boundaries, and confidentiality. An example of this would be a clinician focused on helping their clients deal with feelings of isolation, anxiety, and often overwhelming stress amid COVID-19, but due to their feelings of disconnection, professional boundaries are broken down. This could manifest in many ways; overuse of self-disclosure, projection, and eliciting empathy may burden the client and interfere with the "safe space" that is central to the integrity of the clinical dyad. Another example may include voyeuristic questioning or an inappropriate interest in irrelevant details of the life of the person in treatment.

When countertransference arises, it has the potential to violate the trust, boundaries, and emotional well-being of the client; therefore, the role of clinical supervision and self-care for the clinician is fundamental. In treatment, revisiting painful memories is often accompanied by a high level of emotional disturbance, which can occur when the individual re-experiences some part of a distressing earlier life experience. When an individual is unable to feel, to express, or to release past pain or trauma, it remains internalized and causes long-term dysregulation in the mind and autonomic nervous system. This work is generally slow and gentle, with a lot of consent-seeking that allows the survivor to go deeper and process their unresolved pain from a more empowered place. This facilitates a gentle process of release and unburdening for the survivor. However, this requires compassionate witnessing from the trauma-informed clinician. As noted by Aafjes-van Doorn et al. (2020), the provision of personal and professional support for clinicians working remotely amid a shared trauma can ameliorate the risk of such issues (O'Shea Brown, 2020). Personal support can take many forms, including engaging in long-term supportive self-analysis. In terms of the professional support needed by clinicians, peer consultation groups and connecting with mentors and other colleagues may provide assistance for therapists during these difficult times (Carter & Barnett, 2014). There are no simple solutions, and every clinician is unique in how they experience and seek out support. Ideally, the clinician can explore many avenues of support before finding a place of safety to identify the roots of their VT and/or countertransference. The unexamined history is doomed for repetition; therefore, taking the time to explore one's own experiences and deeply rooted beliefs can expediently enhance clinical practice over the course of a lifetime. In short, going to a clinician who does not examine their own history is like going to a dentist who does not floss. We as clinicians have an ethical responsibility to lead by example and model compassionate witnessing of our past and present lives so that we can show up for others.

Summary

Many clinicians enter into the profession to compassionately witness, heal, and affirm their clients due to their own lived experiences of trauma. Without adequate use of clinical supervision, professional boundaries, and self-care, repeated exposure to trauma can be precarious to the clinician's well-being, causing retraumatization or compassion fatigue. Vicarious trauma refers to the experience of indirect trauma such as the clinician's continuous emotional engagement with a client's traumatic material. This can create cognitive distortions and changes in core belief systems of the clinician, which, in turn, can adversely impact overall functioning and emotional well-being. Furthermore, according to Figley (1995), compassion fatigue refers to reactions that emerge from the trauma clinician's overexposure to client suffering over extended periods of time. Absorbing and compassionately witnessing the emotional weight of trauma survivors' experiences can, over time, negatively impact both the professional identity and personal life of the trauma clinician. If unnoticed, this can lead to ethical dilemmas in the clinical dyad pertaining to self-disclosure, professional boundaries, and lapses in confidentiality. The provision of personal and professional support for clinicians working remotely amid a shared trauma can ameliorate the risk of such issues. Personal support can take many forms, including engaging in long-term supportive self-analysis or sourcing external clinical supervision. However, compassionate witnessing and connection are at the very heart of trauma treatment, and one must care for themselves so that they can adequately show up for their clients.

Questions and Activities for Discussion and Further Reflection

1. Can you define the following terms: (i) vicarious trauma, (ii) secondary traumatic stress, and (iii) shared trauma?
2. Assignment: Write a short reflective essay on how you believe your personal countertransference has impacted your practice to date.
3. Class Discussion Prompt: If unnoticed, countertransference and vicarious trauma (VT) can lead to ethical dilemmas in the clinical dyad pertaining to self-disclosure, professional boundaries, and confidentiality. Discuss the following in smaller groups:

   - How would you respond if you noticed VT and countertransference affecting your clinical practice?
   - What are risks to the client?
   - How would this impact the clinician's assessment and treatment skills?
   - How could supervision be helpful in this instance?
   - How can this be prevented?
   - What would you do if you noticed a colleague's work were being impacted by the above?

References

Asfjes-van Doorn, K., Békés, V., Prout, T. A., & Hoffman, L. (2020). Psychotherapists' vicarious traumatization during the COVID-19 pandemic. *Psychological Trauma: Theory, Research, Practice, and Policy, 12*(S1), S148–S150.

Altman, N., & Davies, J. M. (2002). Out of the blue: Reflections on shared trauma. *Psychoanalytic Dialogues, 12*(3), 359–360.

Berzoff, J., & Kita, E. (2010). Compassion fatigue and countertransference: Two different concepts. *Clinical Social Work Journal, 38*, 341–349. https://doi.org/10.1007/s10615-010-0271-8

Braun, B. G. (1986). Issues in the psychotherapy of multiple personality disorder. In B. G. Braun (Ed.), *Treatment of multiple personality disorder* (pp. 1–28). Washington, DC: American Psychiatric Press.

Carter, L., & Barnett, J. (2014). *Self-care for clinicians in training: A guide to psychological wellness for graduate students in psychology*. Oxford, UK: Oxford University Press.

Courtois, C. (2010). *Healing the incest wound: Adult survivors in therapy* (2nd ed.). New York, NY: Norton.

Eidelson, R., D'Alessio, G., & Eidelson, J. (2003). The impact of September 11 on psychologists. *Professional Psychology: Research and Practice, 34*(2), 144–150.

Figley, C. (1995). *Compassion fatigue: Coping with secondary traumatic stress in those who treat the traumatized*. New York, NY: Brunner/Mazel.

Figley, C. R. (2002). Compassion fatigue: Psychotherapists' chronic lack of self care. *Journal of Clinical Psychology, 58*, 1433–1441. https://doi.org/10.1002/jclp.10090

O'Shea Brown, G. (2020). Internal family systems informed eye movement desensitization and reprocessing: An integrative technique for treatment of complex posttraumatic stress disorder. *International Body Psychotherapy Journal, 19*(2).

O'Shea Brown, G. (2021). Reflections on providing virtual eye movement desensitization and reprocessing therapy in the wake of COVID-19: Survival through adaptation. In C. Tosone (Ed.), *Shared trauma, shared resilience during a pandemic: Social work in the time of COVID-19*. Cham, Switzerland: Springer.

Pearlman, L., & Saakvitne, K. (1995). Trauma and the therapist: Countertransference and vicarious traumatization in psychotherapy with incest survivors. *American Journal of Clinical Hypnosis, 38*(4), 298–299.

Siegfried, C. (2008, March). *Child welfare work and secondary traumatic stress. Child welfare trauma training toolkit: Secondary traumatic stress* (Module 6, Activity 6c). The National Child Traumatic Stress Network.

Saakvitne, K. (2002). Shared trauma: The therapist's increased vulnerability. *Psychoanalytic Dialogues, 12*(3), 443–449.

Stamm, B., Varra, E., Pearlman, L., & Giller, E. (2002). *The helper's power to heal and to be hurt—Or helped—By trying*. Washington, DC: Register Report: A Publication of the National Register of Health Service Providers in Psychology.

Tosone, C., & Bialkin, L. (2003). The impact of mass violence and secondary trauma in clinical practice. In L. A. Straussner & N. Phillips (Eds.), *Social work with victims of mass violence* (pp. 157–167). New York, NY: Jossey Bass.

Tosone, C., Bialkin, L., Campbell, M., Charters, M., Gieri, K., Gross, S., et al. (2003). Shared trauma: Group reflections on the September 11th disaster. *Psychoanalytic Social Work, 10*(1), 57–77.

Tosone, C. (2006). Therapeutic intimacy: A post-9/11 perspective. *Smith College Studies in Social Work, 76*(4), 89–98.

Tosone, C., Nuttman-Shwartz, O., & Stephens, T. (2012). Shared trauma: When the professional is personal. *Clinical Social Work Journal, 40*, 231–239. https://doi.org/10.1007/s10615-012-0395

Chapter 12
Conclusion

Complex trauma is insidious and pervasive in our society; it changes the way an individual perceives themselves and others, in addition to adversely impacting how safe and secure they feel in navigating the world around them. There is a particular veil of shame and secrecy that surrounds complex trauma; however, it is hoped that its formal recognition will shine a light for those suffering in silence. After decades of diligent effort from Herman (1992), van der Kolk, McFarlane, and Weisaeth (1996), and others, complex posttraumatic stress disorder (C-PTSD) was finally included as a diagnostic entity in the *International Classification of Diseases, 11th revision* (*ICD-11*). Endorsement of the *ICD-11* definition of C-PTSD will come into effect on January 1, 2022, almost 30 years after the seminal work of Judith Herman, MD. Herman (1992) proposed that the definition of posttraumatic stress disorder (PTSD) accepted at that time was neither adequate nor appropriate to characterize the complex symptomatology experienced by survivors of prolonged and repeated traumatic events in the formative years. The differentiation of PTSD and C-PTSD is crucial for both theoretical and clinical reasons. The endorsement date of *ICD-11's* definition of C-PTSD will mark three decades during which C-PTSD had been identified but was not officially codified in any diagnostic nomenclature. From a scientific standpoint, nomenclature is regarded as crucial to precision, accuracy, and classification; without clearly determined symptom clusters, the descriptions of the disorder varied. Research on the impacts and treatment of C-PTSD was adversely impacted by the lack of clear diagnostic criteria.

In terms of future research, a clear definition of C-PTSD as a distinct disorder will enhance researchers' capacity to focus on the development of studies to inform identification of risk factors and etiology (Böttche et al., 2018). Clearly defining and recognizing C-PTSD also has clinical implications. Reliable and valid diagnoses

The original version of this chapter was revised. The incorrect author name and affiliation has been removed. The correction to this chapter is available at https://doi.org/10.1007/978-3-030-61416-4_13

G. O'Shea Brown, *Healing Complex Posttraumatic Stress Disorder*, Essential Clinical Social Work Series, https://doi.org/10.1007/978-3-030-61416-4_12

are essential for the measurement and assessment of treatment outcomes, as symptoms associated with C-PTSD require different treatment approaches (Böttche et al., 2018). Past research has found that the treatment of complex trauma should be phase-oriented, multimodal, and skill-focused, with a core emphasis on symptom relief and functional improvement (Briere & Scott, 2006; Courtois, Ford, & Cloitre, 2009). This is to create stabilization and relief to disturbances in self-regulation and interpersonal functioning associated with C-PTSD (WHO, 2018). With the establishment of the *ICD-11* definition of C-PTSD, it is hoped that future research will clearly evaluate and appraise the best practice guidelines covering the causes, symptom presentation, and treatment of C-PTSD. At this juncture, the *Diagnostic and Statistical Manual of Mental Disorders* (DSM) does not formerly recognize C-PTSD as a diagnosis. However, it is hoped that this will follow the lead of the *ICD-11* and will shift toward recognizing C-PTSD and providing clear nomenclature and diagnostic criteria.

With these changes, we may greatly advance our transition to a more trauma-conscious society, in other words, a society that affirms and validates that pervasive childhood abuse and neglect is a deeply wicked problem with significant, long-term repercussions for individuals and society at large. With that, we can begin to acknowledge that prolonged and repeated trauma in the formative years must be prevented rather than treated and pledge ourselves to that goal. The way forward lies not just in enhancing treatment outcomes for complex trauma but also in eradicating complex trauma through preventative practices.

The principle of restoring human connection and agency remains central to the processes of preventing and healing complex trauma. Empowerment and reconnection are the core experiences of recovery. We should not underestimate the healing power of a warm, nurturing presence and the role of the empathic witness as a beacon of hope in the desolate experience of complex trauma. I hope this book has offered you an intimate look at how complex trauma informs the identity, behavior, and thought patterns of survivors. As we work toward becoming a society that is more thoughtful and conscious of the remnants of the childhood experience, it is hoped that advancements in early childhood intervention programs, adequate provisions of mental health services, and equality of access to education and employment will evolve. Survivors of childhood trauma are burdened with significant adversity into adulthood: Adverse childhood experiences are highly correlated to serious problems including lower school achievement, higher rates of criminal behavior, chronic disease, and addiction. The ability to respond to life's challenges in a positive, adaptive manner is rooted in the quality of the relationships that children have with their primary caregivers and other important individuals in their lives. Understanding the importance of this influence emerges directly from an understanding of how much responsiveness facilitates cognitive, social, and emotional development, which enhance one's capacity to adapt to survive in the face of hardship.

Around the world, prisoners of childhood are confined to situations where they feel trapped, powerless, and isolated. In writing *Healing Complex Posttraumatic Stress Disorder: A Clinician's Guide*, it has been my aspiration to integrate the accumulated wisdom and findings of the many clinicians, researchers, and political activists who have worked diligently to prove and attest to the psychological effects of complex trauma and create a body of knowledge that ultimately led to the recognition of C-PTSD in the *ICD-11*. It is my sincere hope that this book has enhanced your understanding of how trauma impacts the mind, body, and brain and of how survivors themselves experience, survive, and heal from trauma.

Though the prevalence and effects of childhood trauma can be disheartening at times, the healing process can positively change the mind, brain, and body. With defined nomenclature and more advanced research, deeper and more meaningful healing can be facilitated by trauma-informed clinicians. Investment in the healthy development of the next generation will continue and build on this pattern, eventually helping to break the cycle of abuse, violence, and trauma.

References

Böttche, M., Ehring, T., Krüger-Gottschalk, A., Rau, H., Schäfer, I., Schellong, J., … Knaevelsrud, C. (2018). Testing the ICD-11 proposal for complex PTSD in trauma-exposed adults: Factor structure and symptom profiles. *European Journal of Psychotraumatology, 9*(1), 1512264. https://doi.org/10.1080/20008198.2018.1512264

Briere, J., & Scott, C. (2006). *Principles of trauma therapy: A guide to symptoms, evaluation, and treatment.* London, UK: Sage.

Courtois, C. A., Ford, J. D., & Cloitre, M. (2009). Best practices in psychotherapy for adults. In C. A. Courtois & J. D. Ford (Eds.), *Treating complex traumatic stress disorders: An evidence-based guide* (pp. 82–103). New York, NY: Guilford Press.

Herman, J. L. (1992). *Trauma and recovery: The aftermath of violence.* New York, NY: Basic Books.

van der Kolk, B. A., McFarlane, A., & Weisaeth, L. (1996). *Traumatic stress.* New York, NY: Guilford Press.

World Health Organization [WHO]. (2018). *The ICD-11 for mortality and morbidity statistics.* Retrieved from https://icd-who-int.proxy.library.nyu.edu/browse11/l-m/en.

Correction to: Conclusion

Correction to:
Chapter 12 in: G. O'Shea Brown, *Healing Complex Posttraumatic Stress Disorder*, Essential Clinical Social Work Series, https://doi.org/10.1007/978-3-030-61416-4_12

The original version of the chapter was inadvertently published with an incorrect author's name and affiliation tagged as "Roman Shvydkoy, Math, Stats, & Comp Sci, University of Illinois at Chicago, Chicago, USA." This has now been corrected as "Gillian O'Shea Brown, New York University, New York, USA."

The updated online version of the chapter can be found at
https://doi.org/10.1007/978-3-030-61416-4_12

G. O'Shea Brown, *Healing Complex Posttraumatic Stress Disorder*, Essential Clinical Social Work Series, https://doi.org/10.1007/978-3-030-61416-4_13

Appendix

The Adult Attachment Interview

The Adult Attachment Interview (AAI) is used to assess to what extent early experiences were characterized by emotional warmth, rejection, neglect, pressure to achieve, or role reversal and, more importantly, the state of mind of the respondent regarding these attachment experiences. The AAI provides a personalized and in-depth insight into trust, vulnerability, relational trauma, and the internal working model. It was developed by psychologists Carol George, PhD; Nancy Kaplan, PhD; and Mary Main, PhD, in 1984. It is a quasi-clinical, semi-structured interview that is generally administered by an AAI-trained clinician to the respondent over the duration of 1 to 2 h.

Training and Certification

Learning to score and code the AAI begins with a 2-week intensive training. As important background, the interview starts with a brief summary of Bowlby's original attachment theory, a description of the Infant Attachment categories of Mary Ainsworth (including the Strange Situation Procedure), and the subsequent links to adult attachment theory and the AAI. Following this preliminary review, the bulk of the training is focused on the AAI scoring and coding system developed by Main and Ruth Goldwyn. AAI transcripts are both studied and scored by trainees outside of class and also carefully reviewed during class time. Less formal discussion of research and clinical questions that arise during the training is scheduled and conducted as needed. Upon completion of the course, trainees are given several booklets to take with them for continued study and practice in preparation for certification testing. The certification process takes an additional 18 months and consists of three tests taken at 6-month intervals. Each test is a set of about ten transcripts to be coded.

For more information on training and certification, please visit attachment-training.com.

G. O'Shea Brown, *Healing Complex Posttraumatic Stress Disorder*, Essential Clinical Social Work Series, https://doi.org/10.1007/978-3-030-61416-4

Trauma-Focused Cognitive Behavioral Therapy

Trauma-Focused Cognitive Behavioral Therapy (TF-CBT) is a skills-based modality used to treat child, adolescent, and adult survivors of trauma, which combines techniques of cognitive behavioral therapy and family therapy. It was first developed in the 1990s by Judith Cohen, MD; Esther Deblinger, PhD; and Anthony Mannarino, PhD, as a modality designed to reduce trauma-related symptomatology. The objective of TF-CBT is to foster the growth of adaptive skills and communication techniques outside of the therapy suite.

Training and Certification

As a graduate student, you will be able to undertake a basic training in this modality. To become certified in TF-CBT, you will be required to have completed a master's or doctoral degree and become a licensed mental health professional. However, graduate students or post-doctoral fellows who have received 2 days of TF-CBT training and at least 12 TF-CBT consultation/supervision sessions from an approved TF-CBT supervisor/trainer will be eligible for certification once they have completed the appropriate requirements and are licensed in their jurisdiction. If you have completed basic training and are seeking to work with a supervisor, please contact the TF-CBT manager at tf-cbt@wpahs.org to ascertain that your instructor has graduated from the TF-CBT train-the-trainer (TTT) program. Upon completion of the hours of consultation, you will be eligible to sit for an exam for licensure.

For more information on Trauma-Focused Cognitive Behavioral Therapy training and certification, please visit tfcbt.org.

Eye Movement Desensitization and Reprocessing

Eye Movement Desensitization and Reprocessing (EMDR) is a therapy modality designed to resolve unprocessed traumatic memories in the body and nervous system, created by Francine Shapiro, PhD, in the 1980s. An EMDRIA-approved EMDR training provides clinicians with the knowledge and skills to utilize EMDR therapy, a comprehensive understanding of case conceptualization and treatment planning, and the ability to integrate EMDR therapy into their clinical practice.

Training and Certification

An EMDRIA-approved EMDR training provides, at a minimum, instruction in the current explanatory model, methodology, and underlying mechanisms of EMDR through lecture, practice, and integrated consultation. All EMDRIA-approved trainings require the minimum of 20 h of supervised practicum and 10 h of clinical consultation. Consultation provides an opportunity for the integration of the theory of EMDR along with the development of EMDR therapy skills. During consultation, trainees receive individualized feedback and instruction in the areas of case conceptualization, client readiness, target selection, treatment planning, specific application of skills, and the integration of EMDR therapy into clinical practice. Consultation is about real cases and not experiences that occur in practicum. EMDRIA-approved EMDR training providers offer different format options; the developer of a specific training may enhance or expand any portion.

EMDR training offered in a university setting usually takes place over an entire (12-week) semester, while trainings offered in a post-graduate training setting may take place over a 2-weekend period or several weeks or may even be specially tailored around a trainee's or agency's work schedule. Clinicians are eligible to become EMDR International Association-certified therapists if they are fully licensed in their mental health professional field for independent practice and have 2 years of experience (minimum) in that field. Specific EMDR requirements include completion of an EMDR International Association-approved training program in EMDR therapy, a minimum of 50 clinical sessions in which EMDR was utilized, and 20 h of consultation in EMDR by an approved consultant or consultant in training (CIT). Please note that a CIT can provide up to 15 h of the required 20 h of consultation for certification. To maintain the credential, EMDR International Association-certified therapists must complete 12 h of continuing education in EMDR every 2 years (Table 1).

For more information on the EMDR Basic Training and Certification, please visit emdria.org.

Internal Family Systems

In 1995, Richard Schwartz, PhD, pioneered the Internal Family Systems (IFS) Model, which applies family systems theory to the integration of sub-personalities or parts of self in order to access an internal self-leadership quality. Trainings are

Table 1 Summary of EMDR basic training and certification

Competency levels	Training requirements	Hours of consultation	Cumulative EMDR clients	Cumulative EMDR sessions	Hours of CIT consultation
EMDR-trained therapist	EMDRIA-approved basic training (Parts 1 and 2)	10			
EMDRIA-certified therapist	Additional 12 EMDRIA-approved CEU hours	Additional 20	25	50	
EMDRIA-approved consultant			75	300	20

Source: emdria.org

through thoughtful application of ego-state-informed language, which can facilitate compassionate, nonjudgmental witnessing of ego parts that are coming to voice so that they can be heard and even unburdened of their fears.

IFS trainings are open to professionals of the mental health community; in addition, others may also participate in IFS trainings, including master's and doctoral students in the healing arts and sciences, pastoral counselors, dance and art therapists, and healthcare professionals in allied field.

Training

IFS Institute offers progressive levels of training in Internal Family Systems, from beginning (Level 1) through advanced (Level 3). Level 1 training occurs over six weekends within a 12-month period; it also can occur in compressed retreat training experiences. Participants need to have successfully completed Level 1 training in order to enroll in a Level 2 training, and those who wish to enroll in a Level 3 training need to have successfully completed a Level 2 program. As a participant in these trainings, you will learn both IFS theory and technique, thus gaining the knowledge and skills you need to understand and actively use IFS with individuals, couples, children, families, and groups.

For more information on the IFS Training, please visit ifs-institute.com.

Sensorimotor Psychotherapy

Sensorimotor Psychotherapy (SP) was developed in the late 1980s by psychologist Pat Ogden, PhD. The theoretical model of SP is built on traditionally accepted therapeutic interventions and neurologically informed trauma research. SP is a somatically oriented talk therapy which approaches affect dysregulation as a subcortical physiological issue central to the treatment of traumatic stress. As SP does not require the use of touch (hands-on intervention), it is a somatic approach which can be integrated into other therapy modalities for trauma-related disorders. SP works to defuse the dysregulated autonomic arousal and support the client in building resources to manage their emotions and process their trauma safely.

Training

The Sensorimotor Psychotherapy Institute offers progressive levels of training in SP, from beginning (Level 1) through advanced (Level 3) in addition to training in Complex Trauma and Dissociation. Level 1 training occurs over ten weekends within a 12-month period. Participants need to have successfully completed Level 1 training in order to enroll in a Level 2 training, and those who wish to enroll in a Level 3 training need to have successfully completed a Level 2 program. Training is open to graduate students and licensed mental health professionals. Candidates who wish to participate in the Training Program must complete an online application, which consists of a questionnaire and the requirement to upload a resume or curriculum vitae (CV), as well as provide proof of one of the following:

- Licensure in a mental health profession

- Legal authorization to practice as a mental health professional in state/province or country of residence
- Enrollment in a graduate-level mental health program at an accredited college or university or post-graduate degree and engagement in the process of qualifying as a mental health professional legally authorized to practice

For more information on the IFS Training, please visit sensorimotorpsychotherapy.org.

Somatic Experiencing

For many trauma survivors, the body can become a source of pain, shame, or intrusion; therefore, locating safety in the body is one of the foundational steps of trauma treatment. Somatic Experiencing (SE) is a body-focused therapy designed by Peter Levine, PhD, over the past 45 years. SE integrates bodily awareness into the psychotherapeutic process as a means to resolve the symptoms of chronic stress and post-traumatic stress.

Training

The Somatic Experiencing® Professional Training is a continuing education certificate program designed to enhance the skills of professionals working with traumatized or stressed individuals. It takes place over the course of 3 years. Participants of the program must be professionals with an active practice so that the techniques learned in the training can be immediately applied and developed throughout the course of the program, although graduate students participating in an internship program may be considered for enrollment. Professionals who may qualify for the SE™ Professional Training program may include:

- Mental Health Professionals: psychologists, psychiatrists, psychoanalysts, psychotherapists, social workers, counselors, marriage and family therapists, expressive arts therapists, etc.
- Medical and Alternative Medicine Professionals: medical doctors, nurses and nurse practitioners, occupational therapists, physical therapists, chiropractors, emergency medical workers, surgeons, obstetricians, midwives, acupuncturists, naturopathic doctors, etc.
- Bodyworkers: massage therapists, Rolfers®, craniosacral and polarity therapists, Feldenkrais practitioners, yoga therapists, etc.
- Others: first responders, crisis center staff, educators, mediators, clergy, chaplains, coaches, etc.

The program is designed to train professionals in working more effectively with client trauma. It is not suitable for those solely seeking a personal growth experience or for those who do not have an active professional practice.

For more information on Somatic Experiencing® International, please visit traumahealing.org.

Index

G. O'Shea Brown, *Healing Complex Posttraumatic Stress Disorder*, Essential Clinical Social Work Series, https://doi.org/10.1007/978-3-030-61416-4

MIX
Papier aus verantwortungsvollen Quellen
Paper from responsible sources
FSC® C105338

If you have any concerns about our products,
you can contact us on
ProductSafety@springernature.com

In case Publisher is established outside the EU,
the EU authorized representative is:
Springer Nature Customer Service Center GmbH
Europaplatz 3, 69115 Heidelberg, Germany

Printed by Libri Plureos GmbH
in Hamburg, Germany